RAPID WEIGHT LOSS HYPNOSIS AND MEDITATION

Daily affirmations and motivation sentences to increase your self-esteem. Fight anxiety and body fat with mind psychology. Gastric band and deep sleep hypnosis.

Table of Contents

PART 1

RAPID WEIGHT LOSS HYPNOSIS

Introduction

There is no denying that obesity and the associated health problems are one of the biggest challenges faced not only by western countries but also in many other developing countries. The Journal of Health Economics provides more than $ 200 billion annually in the United States for medical obesity research costs. According to SAD (Standard American Diet), processed foods and beverages high in fat, sodium, and sugar that are spread to other countries increase heart disease, diabetes, and other life-threatening problems. The food industry has been treating overweight people for decades (more than $ 2 billion in the U.S. alone in 2015) - most people have tried various diets and other programs that either fail or work temporarily and have made them even more discouraged.

You will find tons of help books that give you diet plans, but they are useless. If you question this, when trying to meet the diet's requirements, let alone allow all of the ingredients, you will lose weight with only the effort required to follow the diet. But here is the most critical statistic that anyone who wants to lose weight should know. Most people who lose weight successfully go on a diet and gain even more weight in the first year! These statistics include people who have participated in The Biggest Loser or whose stomachs have been stapled. This is the most suppressed statistic in the food industry: only 3 in 100 people who reach their goal manage to maintain this weight loss beyond the first year.

A post-mortem with the rest of the 97 people who struggled to keep their weight down showed that they were much hungry after trying their regular diet again than they were before the weight loss program. They have been busy eating since the end of their diet, and some are crazy about food.

From the perspective of human evolution, eating is the phenomenon of the last second. Historically telling, the 1920s was a mere failure to promote less eating, but as a society, the cycle of dietary habits that triggered famine brain mechanisms began until the late 1960s.

A weight reduction diet, by definition, requires a decrease in food admission underneath what the body needs to keep up its present shape. There is no genuine food lack, however all the inherent instruments that guarantee our record endurance fat misfortune. This decrease actuates a neural circuit that utilizes a lot of hormones that cause inordinate utilization of food. This component is just called hunger.

Unreasonable utilization goes about as the mind's fundamental prize framework for diet. Shockingly, scientists have found that weight reduction of various sorts utilizes our neurochemical weapons. On the chance that you have a lot of fat, your body won't know it. He possibly "knows" on the off chance that you are in danger of losing fat. In a valiant exertion to recover homeostasis, our framework decreases the degrees of satiety-showing hormones (leptin and insulin) and draws the fasting hormone "ghrelin" into the circulation system. This hormone brings about an expanded want for food that prompts extra calorie consumption and, eventually, further weight gain.

Researchers are not yet mindful of how the cerebrum and the normal starvation framework collaborate to help or stay away from one another. What we can be sure of is that numerous customary weight control plans lead to a psyche fixated on food. Accordingly, the foundation of the issue lies in the cerebrum where this cycle proceeds. The way we can save us from this cycle is to optimize brain activity. This optimization and control are what you will learn in this guidebook. Thankfully, we can change our brain patterns to behave differently. In this guidebook, we will study self-hypnosis, cognitive behavioral therapy, sleep learning system, and meditation to control our brain and overcome food cravings. To simply put, we will optimize the brain activity.

How Does the Mind Work?

They say we only use about 10% of our brains. That may be real, but I'd rather look at it differently. Consider 10 percent of your conscious mind. In other words, that part generates what you want, the part that thinks about you, analyzes what's going on, makes decisions and is your will power. So, it's a powerful mind pair.

But where's the mind's other 90%? Imagine the subconscious part. It's different from the conscious component. It doesn't think so. This holds all of your ideals, convictions, behaviors, history, and much more. That's the mental part that really regulates you.

Once you've learned to ride a bike and balanced, you'll never forget. If you haven't been on for a while, you may be out of practice, but once you get on your subconscious, you get into gear, and you're able to balance and ride really quickly.

The subconscious is computer-like. When you've programmed it, you'll get what you put in it. When your subconscious mind is full of trash and things you don't like, then that's what it's going to give you. It doesn't think eating when you're full is evil. It's just because, in the past, you designed it that way.

If the subconscious is about 90% of the mind and therefore stronger, why does it not respond to what the imaginative analytical conscious mind says? It's all about what you know and says it. Imagine a 7-year-old. She can be really supportive, or she can dig her heels down, not do what you want, and ignore you. When she's supportive, your mind's open to new ideas and improvement. Yet when she's unhelpful, avoiding the negative situation, that's different. When you try to tell her what you want, she'll probably forget you. When you try to push her to listen, it won't work either.

And how can you make changes to the subconscious? I use self-hypnosis myself, but if you haven't mastered it yet, you can use an affirmation instead. An affirmation is a constructive message you like. When you repeat an affirmation several times out loud, and to yourself, then the subconscious can note and take in what you affirm.

To make the affirmation function better and improve your mind's strength, you should do two things:

- Make sure the affirmation has some value for you. When you have eating disorders, and you make an affirmation, "I'm in control of my weight," the subconscious will forget the affirmation because it's not real. However, if you said, "I get more control of my eating habits every day," then work is more likely.
- Put as an issue. If you are seeking confirmation, the mind must first take it and find out what it means before it's real. It already starts after the affirmation and is real for you.

Conscious Mind and Subconscious Mind

Conscious Mind

The conscious mind can be compared to a word processor. It is the decision-maker for our day to day chores. This "processor" sends programs to the subconscious mind to perform certain tasks, observes how subconscious programs perform them, and then decides what else needs to be done.

The conscious mind is estimated to be only 12% of our minds. What it perceives as a belief is not exactly what our subconscious believes. You may think that there is absolutely no limitation in the subconscious for an issue, but they may still be there.

A unique quality of the conscious mind is that it can quickly judge what is right and what is wrong, something that the subconscious does not do. The conscious decide which information should be kept in the brain and which should not.

Subconscious Mind

This mind is like a system hard disk. It contains memories, habits, beliefs, self-image and controls autonomous bodily functions. It is both the deposit of information and the executors of the tasks. It also contains "pre-defined instructions" that we don't have to consciously think about, such as keeping our heart beating, our breathing, our digestion ...

The subconscious is estimated to be 88% of the mind. This means that when we recognize that one of our beliefs is negative, 12% of our mind wants to change the other 88%. Any decision to change is formed mainly in our conscious mind. This decision will, in some way, conflict with existing beliefs.

The subconscious mind's strength is incredible. By knowing the power of the inner mind, people can alter their unhappy life aspects. The subconscious mind occupies nearly all minds by about 88 percent. If people learn how to manage this subconscious mind properly, they can do everything in life. Your subconscious mind component represents personal patterns, temperament, and memory. And if you're looking for a positive shift of attitudes, actions or memory, then you have to focus on the subconscious mind.

The mind is closely associated with our experience, and it can show in the form of mental or physical disorder if we feed negative thoughts. Not letting negative thoughts spread in the subconscious mind. The future relies on people's thoughts and beliefs. If a person wants to win, they must have a winning attitude. Only then will they accomplish other things in life. It also gives positive inputs for positive output. Ignore negative thoughts because your subconscious mind cannot distinguish the difference between good or bad. So, thrive with good thoughts to increase the mind's healing power. Meditation and relaxation can effectively regulate the body.

Individuals can connect quickly with their subconscious mind using powerful affirmations. Affirmation is just constant reinforcement of optimistic thoughts. And it's really important to direct the good aspects. Through adding the strength of affirmations, people will strengthen their subconscious influence and boost enormous quantities of ability they never knew they had. And whatever the mind thinks it can do. Therefore, hitting the part of the subconscious mind may be a better way to expose the latent ability of the mind. So, if people keep saying good thoughts constantly and holding faith in subconscious forces, they easily resolve their pain and hard times and pull circumstances that will make this conviction come true.

Subconscious mind strength is always misunderstood because people do not recognize their virtues. The part of the subconscious mind is the storage bank of all reinforcement (good or bad) we obtain in our surroundings. In adolescence, this affirmation directly affects one's behaviors. These same patterns decide our personality. To enhance our mind's capacity, feeding the right affirmation (repeatedly) into the subconscious is very necessary. This is possible with subliminal contact. People may write a tailor-made text message denoting positive affirmation. The encouragement is directed at the subconscious mind to develop a new habit. With age, developing new habits is extremely difficult for an aged person. Subliminal messaging can frame new habits.

All of these allow for versatility to adapt to new behaviors. If properly used, the subconscious mind has forces far beyond human understanding. Uncover subconscious mind control by subliminal messaging.

Ways to Use the Power of Your Mind to Increase Your Well-Being

We all want to feel good, love, have good jobs, etc. Those aspects are what most people around the world call "the good life." Though we all realize that being loved will not always make us feel good. This essay will explore the relationship between how we use our minds' strength and sense of well-being.

Well-being is not about physical comfort, but rather the far more profound concept of living a life that has a purpose, fulfilling your potential, or knowing how you make a positive difference in the world. People working in health care have a good attitude towards life in describing well-being as proof that we care for ourselves.

The "power of the mind" requires more than mental energy. Rather, it is a holistic concept that includes: 1) our being conscious and linked to the life force, 2) tracking minute emotional reactions to what is occurring at the moment, with the ability to 3) see, guide, and often direct our actions in the direction we believe would lead us to a more fulfilling existence. It may be more appropriate to suggest that the power of our minds is our intellectual capacity to interpret and bring awareness to our existence as linked to the world around us — meaning that we are steering the ship, but it is also linked to the wider network of existence.

And what should we do to use the strength inherent in this holistic view of mind control to improve our well-being?

What Is Hypnosis?

As indicated by specialists, hypnosis is viewed as a condition of cognizance that includes the engaged consideration alongside the diminished fringe mindfulness that is described by the member's expanded ability to react to recommendations that are given. This implies the member will enter an alternate perspective and will be substantially more defenseless to following the recommendations that are given by the trance inducer.

It is broadly perceived that two hypothesis bunches help to depict what's going on during the hypnosis time frame. The first is the changing state hypothesis. The individuals who follow this hypothesis see that hypnosis resembles a daze or a perspective that is adjusted where the member will see that their mindfulness is, to some degree, not quite the same as what they would see in their common cognizant state. The other hypothesis is non-state speculations. The individuals who follow this hypothesis don't believe that the individuals who experience hypnosis are going into various conditions of awareness. Or maybe, the member is working with the subliminal specialist to enter a sort of inventive job authorization.

While in hypnosis, the member is thought to have more fixation and center that couples together with another capacity to focus on a particular memory or thought strongly. During this procedure, the member is likewise ready to shut out different sources that may be diverting to them. The mesmerizing subjects are thought to demonstrate an increased capacity to react to recommendations that are given to them, particularly when these proposals originate from the subliminal specialist. The procedure that is utilized to put the member into hypnosis is knitted hypnotic enlistment and will include a progression of proposals and guidelines that are utilized as a kind of warm-up.

There is a wide range of musings that are raised by specialists with regards to what the meaning of hypnosis is. The wide assortment of these definitions originates from the way that there are simply such huge numbers of various conditions that accompany hypnosis, and nobody individual has a similar encounter when they are experiencing it.

Some various perspectives and articulations have been made about hypnosis. A few people accept that hypnosis is genuine and are suspicious that the legislature and others around them will attempt to control their minds. Others don't have faith in hypnosis at all and feel that it is only skillful deception. No doubt, the possibility of hypnosis as mind control falls someplace in the center.

There are three phases of hypnosis that are perceived by the mental network. These three phases incorporate acceptance, recommendation, and defenselessness. Every one of them is critical to the hypnosis procedure and will be talked about further underneath.

Induction

The principal phase of hypnosis is induction. Before the member experiences the full hypnosis, they will be acquainted with the hypnotic enlistment method. For a long time, this was believed to be the strategy used to place the subject into their hypnotic stupor. However, that definition has changed some in current occasions. A portion of the non-state scholars has seen this stage somewhat in an unexpected way. Rather they consider this to be as the strategy to elevate the

Members' desires for what will occur, characterizing the job that they will play, standing out enough to be noticed to center the correct way, and any of the different advances that are required to lead the member into the correct heading for hypnosis.

There are a few induction procedures that can be utilized during hypnosis. The most notable and compelling strategies are Braid's "eye obsession" method or "Braidism." There are many varieties of this methodology, including the Stanford Hypnotic Susceptibility Scale (SHSS). This scale is the most utilized instrument to examine in the field of hypnosis.

To utilize the Braid enlistment procedures, you should follow several means. The first is to take any object that you can find that is brilliant, for example, a watch case, and hold it between the centers, fore, and thumb fingers on the left hand. You will need to hold this item around 8-15 crawls from the eyes of the member. Hold the item someplace over the brow, so it creates a ton of strain on the eyelids and eyes during the procedure with the goal that the member can keep up a fixed gaze on the article consistently.

The trance inducer should then disclose to the member that they should focus their eyes consistently on the article. The patient will likewise need to concentrate their mind on that specific item. They ought not to be permitted to consider different things or let their minds and eyes meander or, in all likelihood, the procedure won't be effective.

A little while later, the member's eyes will start to enlarge. With somewhat more time, the member will start to accept a wavy movement. If the member automatically shuts their eyelids when the center and forefingers of the correct hand are conveyed from the eyes to the item, at that point, they are in the stupor. If not, at that point, the member should start once more; make a point to tell the member that they are to permit their eyes to close once the fingers are conveyed in a comparable movement back towards the eyes once more. This will get the patient to go into the adjusted perspective that is knaps hypnosis.

While Braid remained by his method, he acknowledged that utilizing the acceptance procedure of hypnosis isn't constantly fundamental for each case. Analysts in current occasions have typically discovered that the acceptance strategy isn't as essential with the impacts of hypnotic recommendation as recently suspected. After some time, different other options and varieties of the first hypnotic acceptance procedure have been created, even though the Braid strategy is as yet thought about the best.

Recommendation

Present-day sleep induction utilizes a variety of proposal shapes to be fruitful, for example, representations, implications, roundabout or non-verbal recommendations, direct verbal proposals, and different metaphors and recommendations that are non-verbal. A portion of the non-verbal proposals that might be utilized during the recommendation stage would incorporate physical manipulation, voice tonality, and mental symbolism.

Something that must be considered concerning hypnosis is the contrast between the oblivious and the cognizant mind. There are a few trance specialists who see the phase of the proposal as a method of conveying that is guided generally to the cognizant mind of the subject. Others in the field will see it the other way; they see the correspondence happening between the operator and the subconscious or oblivious mind.

They accepted that the recommendations were being tended to directly to the conscious piece of the subject's mind, as opposed to the oblivious part. Braid goes further and characterizes the demonstration of trance induction as the engaged consideration upon the proposal or the

18

predominant thought. The fear of a great many people that subliminal specialists will have the option to get into their oblivious and cause them to do and think things outside their ability to control is inconceivable as per the individuals who follow this line of reasoning.

The idea of the mind has additionally been the determinant of the various originations about the recommendation. The individuals who accepted that the reactions given are through the oblivious mind, for example, on account of Milton Erickson, raise the instances of utilizing aberrant recommendations. Huge numbers of these aberrant proposals, for example, stories or representations, will shroud their expected importance to cover it from the cognizant mind of the subject. The subconscious recommendation is a type of hypnosis that depends on the hypothesis of the oblivious mind. If the oblivious mind were not being utilized in hypnosis, this sort of recommendation would not be conceivable. The contrasts between the two gatherings are genuinely simple to perceive; the individuals who accept that the recommendations will go fundamentally to the cognizant mind will utilize direct verbal guidelines and proposals while the individuals who accept the proposals will go essentially to the oblivious mind will utilize stories and analogies with concealed implications.

In both of these hypotheses of figured, the member should have the option to concentrate on one article or thought. This permits them to be driven toward the path that is required to go into the hypnotic state. When the recommendation stage has been finished effectively, the member will, at that point, have the option to move into the third stage, powerlessness.

Powerlessness

After some time, it has been seen that individuals will respond contrastingly to hypnosis. A few people find that they can fall into a hypnotic stupor reasonably effectively and don't need to apply a lot of energy into the procedure by any means. Others may find that they can get into the hypnotic daze, however, simply after a drawn-out timeframe and with some exertion. Still, others will find that they can't get into the hypnotic stupor, and significantly after proceeding with endeavors, won't arrive at their objectives. One thing that specialists have discovered intriguing about the weakness of various members is that this factor stays steady. If you have had the option to get into a hypnotic perspective effectively, you are probably going to be a similar path for an incredible remainder. Then again, if you have consistently experienced issues in arriving at the hypnotic state and have never been entranced, at that point, almost certainly, you never will.

There have been a few distinct models created after some time to attempt to decide the defenselessness of members to hypnosis. A portion of the more established profundity scales attempted to construe which level of a daze the member was in through the discernible signs that were accessible. These would incorporate things, for example, the unconstrained amnesia. A portion of the more present-day scales works to quantify the level of self-assessed or watched responsiveness to the particular recommendation tests that are given, for example, the immediate proposals of unbending arm nature.

As per the examination that has been finished by Deirdre Barrett, there are two kinds of subjects that are considered profoundly vulnerable to the impacts of subliminal therapy. These two gatherings incorporate dissociates and fantasizers. The fantasizers will score high on the assimilation scales, will have the option to effortlessly shut out the boosts of this present reality without the utilization of hypnosis, invest a great deal of their energy wandering off in fantasy land, had fanciful companions when they were a youngster, and experienced childhood in a situation where nonexistent play was energized.

How Does Hypnosis Work?

I just showed you a breakdown of the phases of hypnosis. But how does hypnosis work? In hypnosis, we can reformulate our unconscious thoughts. You may wonder: why is the hypnotized mind so suggestible? What happens in the brain when we are hypnotized? Can everyone be hypnotized? The short answer is we can likely all be hypnotized!

According to research, the majority of people, about 75-85 percent, can achieve a slight trance. And most of these people share some common traits such as:

- Daydream often
- Get absorbed in daily activities quickly.
- Show more empathy
- Are open-minded about hypnosis.

How to Use Hypnosis to Transform and Re Program Your Mind?

Healing the Body with Hypnosis

Hypnosis is a practice used for losing weight, but since healing forms an essential part of retraining both the body and mind to perform in perfect harmony, it needs to be treated as a tool to calm the mind. Once you've mastered the art of self-control, you can move on and easily convince yourself that you are capable of losing weight, reaching your goal weight, and achieving many other fitness goals that you once thought wasn't possible.

Losing weight is a time-consuming process. The higher weight you have to lose, the more patience and persistence you need to become successful. In that same breath, if you've got a lot of weight to lose, it's most likely that you will also have to address certain health issues. Integrating hypnosis into your daily routine can reduce stress and help obtain a sense of regularity and balance, which is required to lose weight. Medically speaking, since hypnosis treats stress too, it is perfect for anyone suffering from obesity, eating disorders, an overactive or underactive thyroid, or anyone who struggles to follow a healthy, balanced diet.

What Hypnosis Feels Like

Imagine that you are watching an exciting action movie. A dangerous group chases the main character. The protagonist is trapped in a building, and the bad guys are waiting for him outside. You have been immersed in the movie when one of your family members asks you to give them a pillow. What do you do? I suppose you will take the pillow and give it to your relative without taking your eyes off the screen. When you are hypnotized, a similar scenario occurs. You focus on the matter intensely, and everything else becomes irrelevant. The greater the focus, the stronger the tendency to follow the suggestions of the therapist.

However, there is a slightly difference between the attention paid during a movie and in hypnosis. People who watch movies profoundly are more inclined not to reply to the questions they are asked; however, the opposite occurs during hypnosis. Why is that? Based on the observation of Freudian psychologists, this happens due to the difference between the phases of human awareness. They believe that there are three layers of human consciousness: precociousness, consciousness, and the unconscious level. These levels are depicted with an analogy. The level of consciousness that is compared to the visible part of an iceberg seeing it from the water surface represents the moments of our awareness about what's happening around us when we are awake (Cherry, 2019).

The Dangerous side of Hypnosis

There are many dangers that you can run into if you try to hypnotize someone without proper training. The truth is, when someone is hypnotized, you are playing with a vulnerable subconscious and without proper training, and you can easily cause permanent damage to their psyche. It is important that you become properly trained and that you truly understand the basics of psychology before you enter the world of hypnotism.

Understanding how the human mind works at its most vulnerable states can help you prevent harming someone long term or causing them to develop fears and phobias that did not previously exist.

The most important thing to put in mind when diving into someone subconscious is that you have the power to open up memories that they are not ready to face yet. This can cause severe emotional trauma to those who are already "mentally vulnerable."

It is wise to screen the people you hypnotize carefully to ensure that they have not endured any childhood trauma. This is because under hypnosis, these memories can become extremely vivid and the subject may not be able to handle the pain associated with the memories you are unknowingly digging up.

What Is Self-Hypnosis?

Self-hypnosis is a term used when you are the one who is hypnotizing yourself in the absence of a hypnotherapist or psychologist. This requires deep concentration and focus to achieve your goals. Like any regular hypnosis, you will need to have goals for yourself when you are performing hypnosis on yourself. The goals might be to control pain, to direct anger, to eliminate bad habits or to help you rid yourself of any excessive stress that you might be under.

This process is performed by those people who are looking at having a control on the decisions that they might have to make in their lives. This process is close to meditation. Only it has better results when compared to meditation.

Self-Hypnosis Advantages

- You take charge of everything.
- You know yourself better than other people.
- You avoid being controlled by someone with ill intentions.
- You prevent being dependent on somebody else so that you can improve yourself.
- You save money when you do things yourself.
- You can perform hypnosis on yourself wherever and whenever you want as opposed to making scheduled appointments with a hypnotist.
- If you understand how hypnosis is done, you will be able to apply it in endless ways.
- You will not be confined to what a hypnotist tells you or what you read in books.
- If you know how to hypnotize yourself, you can also do it to others.

Self-Hypnosis Disadvantages

- You may be limited by your biases
- You may miss out some things that you are unconsciously or deliberately avoiding
- You may find it cumbersome to comply to your own suggestions especially if you're used to following other people's orders
- You might resist yourself especially if you have self-esteem issues

- You are responsible for the results, so you need to study how it's done instead of relying on someone else to do the hard work for you

If you are looking at performing hypnosis on yourself, ensure that you in your most comfortable clothing. You have to remember that you will need to focus on relaxing yourself. So, it is best if you wear clothes that are loose. You should not be in clothes that will hinder your ability to breathe freely.

The first step to performing self – hypnosis is to prepare yourself mentally. This is, in fact, the main and most important step of the process.

Next, you will need to ensure that you are dressed in your most comfortable attire.

The following step for you is to check the environment that you are in. Check the temperature and the humidity in your surroundings. Humid surroundings are not conducive to performing a self – hypnosis. If you find that the environment suits your needs, but the weather is cold, you can cover yourself with a blanket or dress in warmer clothes and if it is too hot, then you can switch on the fan or air conditioner.

It is of utmost importance that you choose the quietest place in your house. You will need to find an environment where you will not be distracted by either internal or external factors. You should also ensure that the place you choose has the perfect place for you to seat yourself in the most comfortable position. There is no necessity for you to sit on the floor and fold your legs.

You can lie down on your bed or sit on your couch. Just ensure that you are not going to fall asleep. If you feel that lying down will force you to sleep, then assume a semi lie down position and seat yourself on a recliner.

Also ensure that you are not crossing your hands or your legs when you are sitting down or lying down. This is to make sure that you do not find yourself feeling cramped due to the position you are in. This process ideally takes a complete half hour. You should keep yourself away from any distractions. The process will not be effective on you if you are constantly distracted by the people or things around you.

It should ideally take you 15 to 20 minutes to complete the process. Initially you might find that you take a longer amount of time to hypnotize yourself. It is alright if you do not master the technique at the earliest.

You are learning and will master it soon. So, do not be depressed if someone else masters the technique in a week and you do not. In fact, you must not even ponder over who is learning it and is picking it up at what rate.

Each person is different from the rest and will take the amount of time that is suited for them.

You will only achieve your purpose if you succeed in your hypnosis and its process.

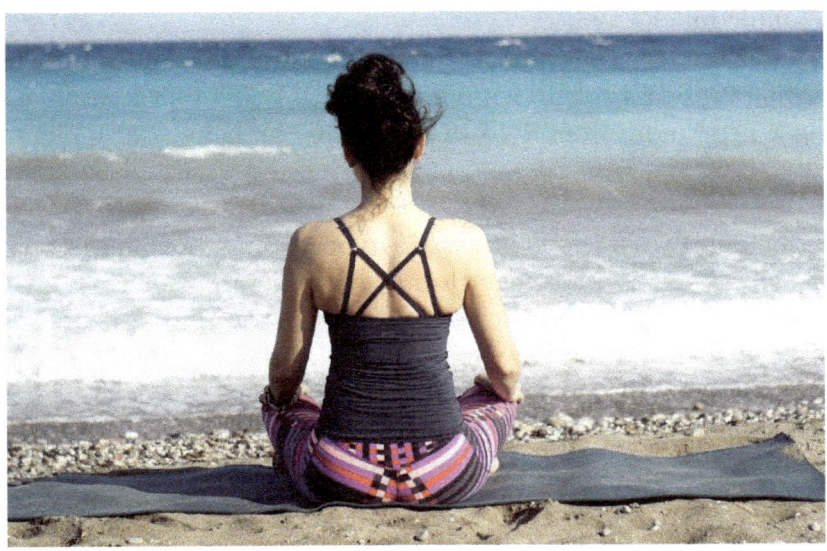

Hypnosis and Weight Loss

One of the most recent forms of hypnosis has something to do with weight loss.

A perfect example of this would be Marion Corns, a woman from the United Kingdom who underwent Hypnosis to believe that she has undergone Gastric Bypass Surgery. By believing in this, she learned how to control the amount she's eating. While she used to eat as many plates of food as she wanted, she now only eats small portions. This is because she believes that her stomach shrunk to the size of a golf ball!

According to her, she has tried a lot of diet plans before but none of them really worked as she would just go back to her old habits, but because she now believes that a gastric bypass has been done, she tells herself not to eat too much anymore.

What's amazing, too, is the fact that she really didn't undergo gastric bypass, and yet, she's able to reap the benefits. An operation would have cost her a little more than $7,000. She didn't actually shelve out that cash, but now, she has lost a lot of pounds—and that's all because of Hypnosis!

She underwent five sessions of gastric hypnosis in a hospital in Spain. She was already supposed to go through the operation there, but then she found out that that the clinic also gives Gastric Hypnosis sessions, so she decided to go for that one. After 5 sessions, she felt like her stomach was tightening, and every time she tries to eat more than she should, she just feels like she's going to throw up.

According to her, what happened was that she went through Cognitive Behavioral Therapy, which could also be a form of hypnosis. Now, she feels like she finally fits in with society, and she no longer feels like she has to hide from people.

Gastric Hypnosis, as well as Weight Loss Hypnosis, in general, is great for overweight teens and adults. It's said that it is now changing the face of weight loss programs not only in the United Kingdom but in the whole world, as well. This is because people learn how to be more disciplined— and they also learn to understand that they can lose weight even without using too much cash, as long as they know how to control themselves.

It's a striking method to hold yourself under tight restraints, and you'll have the option to lose a couple of additional pounds while as yet attempting to keep your body fit as a fiddle. It's proper on the off chance that you do this with an eating regimen and exercise schedule, for it'll permit you to improve and accomplish more outcomes.

Hypnosis is not a miraculous cure to weight problems. It is actually a complex process. For instance, you cannot just hypnotize someone into eating less. If that person eats less, then his energy would drop. He'd have less energy to move about. If he isn't physically active, his metabolism will be at risk of slowing down, which will eventually result in the body burning lesser amount of fat. It's counterproductive since one has to lose fat in order to lose unwanted weight. Hypnosis for weight loss requires an overall approach.

Is Hypnosis Effective for Weight Loss?

Because hypnosis can affect a person's unconscious motivations, patterns, and feelings, it can be used effectively to help someone who deals with weight problems. The key is to change the way of thinking. For instance, we eat because food tastes good and because it is necessary for survival. However, we often forget about the importance of eating mindfully and healthily. When we begin to feel that we want to consume food in a healthy manner then it will change everything.

Hypnosis works in a way that it can be used to help someone naturally feel that he is making the right choice when it comes to food. Does this mean take away someone's willpower? It doesn't. What it simply means is helping someone feel better about using his willpower as far as food choices are concerned.

Losing weight, after all, is not about getting rid of something we do not want or need. People have become so focused on exercise routines and obsessed with 'healthy' foods. It is of course, perfectly alright to pay attention to these things but it is also important to train our brains. That is where hypnosis comes in.

Hypnosis can help in such a way that a person can create a new relationship with his body and with food. Rather than taking away someone's willpower, hypnosis can be used successfully to reinforce someone's power to choose and be more honest with these choices. For instance, you know you can always have chocolate cake and you can have as much as you want but do you really have to have it? You know you want it, but do you really need it?

There are various approaches to using hypnosis for weight loss. Do not simply focus on one aspect. Choose a set of approaches relevant to that person.

- Use suggestions to help the person envision the body he wants and the level of health and fitness he wants to achieve.
- Encourage the person to level up his fat-burning metabolism. Provide certain cues that will remind him to exercise. For instance, you can suggest that at a specific time of each day, his legs will feel restless, which means it is time to exercise.

- Metaphors can also be used successfully. For example, you can conjure up an image in the person's mind of a sculptor facing a shapeless rock. In order to uncover the real form of that rock, the sculptor must work on it little by little, carefully and patiently. When the real form is revealed, he can get rid of the excess and needless rocks.
- Another imagery you can use to help someone lose weight is to guide him into visualizing that he is wearing a fat suit. Guide him into imagining that he is able to discard layers from his fat suit. Reinforce that feeling of relief as he removes one layer at a time until the suit is in the 'right' size, the way he wants his body to look like.
- Help the person focus not just on numbers and weight but also on health and fitness.
- Help the person make a distinction between real food and fake food, the ones that are good for him and the ones that aren't.
- Use disassociation to help this person see himself in the future when he eats well, exercises regularly, looking slimmer and feeling much lighter.
- Use age progression. Take him into the future where he has become slimmer. Suggest that he goes back in time from the future and remember exactly what he needed to do to make this happen and how easy and effortless it was.
- Help him remember that when he feels the desire to eat unhealthily or consume food when he is not hungry, he is not reaching his goal. Let him imagine how it will make him feel not to reach his goal.

What is Hypnosis for Weight Loss?

It's primarily using hypnosis procedures to allow you to lose weight. It's a way to lose a few more pounds. But most of the time, it is paired with a diet strategy. It is commendable that you continue a good regimen of food, followed by mild exercise. But, this will allow you to shed weight faster, and if you're someone who has cravings for things, then this will help you.

It's also a part of the advice that people do get. You'll be able to get help on your issues pertaining to food, and this form of hypnosis will allow you to have a great time with your yearnings. You can do this with an expert, but you can also do it yourself. It'll allow you rule your life, and you'll control those bad yearnings you have.

How Hypnosis Can Help You Lose Weight

The way it works is simple. When you use hypnosis, you are in a state of satiety and concentration. He's also in a very relaxed and implicit state, so what they tell him is basically taken in a real way. You will use mental images to interpret the meaning of the spoken words. You will focus your attention on this and when your mind is in a unifying state, it will begin to make your subconscious handle your desires. It's an amazing way to stay in control, and you can lose a few extra pounds while trying to keep your body in shape. It is better to do this with a diet and exercise program, as it will allow you to overcome it better and achieve more results.

It is best to do this when you have time to deal with this problem. You will need at least thirty minutes of silence to handle these desires, ideally a maximum of one hour. It will handle some very serious problems, so make sure you are relaxed and able to get back to reality before and after hypnosis improves you.

The Benefits

There are other benefits of using hypnosis for weight loss. The obvious big one is that you lose weight. That's the one people will notice. You'll start to shed those pounds, and you might lose more than you expected. It won't be significant, such as like fifty pounds or more, but if you want to help your body and allow yourself the benefits of being able to control the cravings to lose weight, then this is perfect for you.

Another benefit that people don't realize is how relaxed you are. You'll actually be able to become more relaxed as a result of this. By relaxing the body, you'll be able also to reduce your blood pressure levels and even stop the risk of heart disease. Hypnosis for weight loss allows you to put yourself in a relaxed state for at least an hour, and when you wake up, you'll feel more relaxed. It can also help with bodily tissues, such as muscle aches and pains. If you want to use this to help with those issues as well, it'll definitely do the trick.

Hypnosis utilizes these proposals and a lot more to assist you with vanquishing your awful dietary patterns. Obviously, not all proposals will apply to everybody. The objective is to make a rest treatment plan, either with the assistance of a rest advisor or all alone, that will incorporate proposals that intrigue you.

Weight reduction hypnosis causes you to consider it beneficial to be as scrumptious. Hypnosis can assist you with seeing a sound eating regimen as agreeable.

Then there are the lasting benefits of it. These are the benefits that you'll get because of the hypnosis. When you're doing this, you'll be able to tackle those parts of your subconscious that think it's okay to eat when you're stressed, or it'll tell you to eat more than necessary. occasionally, your mind can be your worst enemy, and this is certainly one of those times. With hypnosis for weight loss, you'll allow yourself to handle your body in a positive manner. If you do this, you'll actually allow yourself to control your cravings and desires through the use of hypnosis. It might seem crazy, but it is possible.

A Basic Self Hypnosis Session for Weight Loss

Sit back, unwind and close your eyes
Feel the pressure on your brow
Feel all the pressure leave.
Feel this unwinding on your brow
Also, in your eyes
Also, presently your eyelids are getting overwhelming
So overwhelming that they would prefer even not to open, they are so loose
They may shudder a bit.
Be that as it may, it's alright...
Feel how overwhelming they are.
Your mouth may even open a little
it's typical...
Unwind with each breath you take,
You're so loosened up now
Progressively loose with every full breath you take.
Deep presently, breathing heavier as you go further and more profound.
Presently envision this...
Envision being in this excellent and beguiling field
At the base of your feet, there is an awesome walkway and block steps
This prompts a sheltered and exceptionally loosening up woods.
These means will take you to a covert government of profound trance.
Get these means together at this point.
While tallying down from 10 to 0
Every difficult will take you more profound and more profound.
Believe it or not, generally excellent; it's going very well at this point.
10: venture out
9: getting further
8: presently down
7: much more profound
6: so magnificently loose
5: Deeper and more profound
4: you are presently entering a condition of profound and profound trance

3: develop

2: so, loosened up that you can even move around, feeling incredibly, good. More agreeable than any time in recent memory, never felt

1: you will enter this delightful spot of harmony and peacefulness called profound and profound entrancing.

0: keeps on going further and more profound, so quiet thus loose; Continue to loosen up presently, breathing effectively and tuning in to light music as you go further and further.

Envision an entryway,

directly before you

It has a positive sign on the entryway.

the positive sign must imply that you enter.

At the point when you open the gateway, you see five stages.

Plunging to a room brimming with dials and meters on all the dividers.

Go down those means

If you don't mind note that all counters and dials appear to proceed inconclusively.

There are such huge numbers of meters and dials

In any case, when you take a gander at them, you notice that they are separately named.

A meter is named "digestion."

The other is named "cholesterol."

Another is named "pulse."

What's more, another named "muscle versus fat and weight."

And keeping in mind that you take a gander at a huge number of meters and quadrants,

You will understand that you are in the control room of your psyche

Sitting in the focal point of this control room is a book called "flawless wellbeing."

It has your name in the book.

Go to that book

Investigate

Look through the words

Start to see that each page has a picture of every quadrant and an arrangement in the quadrant.

What speaks to consummate wellbeing for you.

Begin looking through the pages

As you look through the book, you see a mirror toward the edge of the room.

You approach the mirror

While you take a gander at yourself in this mirror

Envision the mirror indicating all the various edges

In this mirror, you see an ideal impression of you with the right weight and size you need to be.

Take a gander at you from all points

With all the bends in the correct spots

Your garments adjust impeccably to your body.

As you take a gander at the genuine excellence of your appearance,

Tune in to your appearance by giving them these recommendations:

Starting now and into the nearest future I will bite my food longer and more slow

Starting now and into the nearest future, when I plunk down to eat.

I will gauge my appetite level on a size of one to ten.

Zero is starving and ten are full to the point that I can't eat another chomp.

Starting now and into the nearest future, I will quit eating at 6 or 7.

Presently I need to eat a new and sound wellspring of vegetables.

Remember that your appearance connects with contact yours,

At the point when his hands come in get in touch with, you feel a genuine wellspring of adoration from your oblivious reflection.

Feel the cozy wellspring of affection immersing your heart

What's more, presently you see your appearance connecting your hand

At the point when you connect with take your appearance.

Venture forward in your appearance as you become your appearance.

Feel that it is so ideal to turn into your appearance

Come out of the mirror into another existence of wellbeing and imperativeness.

Return to your ideal wellbeing control room

Permit yourself to make sheltered and moderate modifications.

Begin causing you to notice the sensations inside your body

As you believe, you start to address.

The truth is out...

Feel the sensations

Feel the ideal weight you need

As your body moves towards flawless size
Accomplishing your ideal weight
I will check from 1 to 4 and thusly, you will wake up.
With each check, you'll ensure these proposals are somewhere down in your oblivious brain:
1: feel great about yourself, at last realizing that you are in charge
2: you need solid nourishments to assist you with gauging your optimal weight
3: prepared currently to take the necessary steps to achieve this and
4: eyes open, completely conscious, splendid and alert, presently completely wakeful.
It's hard to believe, but it's true...
A More Advanced Self Hypnosis Session
If you don't mind, make yourself agreeable
Settle in...
Try not to stress over how profoundly you loosen up you are and go into a daze
You don't need to attempt.
Simply tune in...
Take a full breath
also, other
Continue seeing your moderate, consistent relaxing
Give close consideration to the inclination that the chest rises and falls
Feel that positive pneumatic force
With the breath coming
As you discharge the air
You can even envision that the air is sheltered,
Recuperating shading when it enters and leaves your body
It likewise directs you to a profoundly loosened up state
Presently you are loose...
Time to treat the piece of you that wouldn't like to get thinner.
Some portion of you can oppose your objective
That is, it...
This piece of you that wouldn't like to get more fit
Presently you can confront that piece of you
Not as a foe or a casualty.
Be that as it may, as a tragically deceased companion

This piece of you that is harmed
Dismissed by others
Dismissed by you
What's more, right now is an ideal advantage to mend.
Presently isn't an ideal opportunity to make harmony within you
Presently you have the chance to accommodate
Gradually, reliably, and effectively arrive at your optimal weight
Allow this to occur...
Let these words hit home as you state you hear them:
I'm sorry you're harmed.
You have been harmed by others.
You have been overlooked by me.
It's an ideal opportunity to recuperate...
I might want you to feel adored.
How about we cooperate
How about we end this war
We can make harmony. It relies upon us.
Envision making harmony with yourself now.
What's more, feel the mending vitality experiencing your body.
By pooling their qualities and assets,
Recuperate your shortcomings and close the hole that has been in your spirit,
It keeps you from completely grasping your most beneficial feeling of self.
You
are a certifiable individual
With every one of your qualities accessible to all pieces of yourself.
Be pleased with yourself
Show yourself in your considerations and sentiments.
You'll before long find all the pieces of yourself that line up with your most advantageous feeling of self
Genuinely, intellectually, inwardly, and profoundly.
Sound food will taste magnificent.
Unfortunate food will taste phony, vacant, and dead.
You will be propelled to move your body.
Welcomes a lively sentiment of general prosperity and wellness.
Feel free to make tranquility within

Remain solid outwardly.

Start to see weight reduction fall into place.

Permit what you realized in this meeting to be coordinated into your being

Also, when you decide to envision yourself before a mirror.

Envision that you are in your preferred outfit.

With the specific weight you need

Feel loose, wakeful and confident.

Envision that your body weight starts to move towards the ideal weight.

Presently take as much time as is needed...

With each tally, you'll ensure these proposals sink somewhere down in your oblivious psyche:

1: see yourself the size and shape you need to be you have the right to be.

2: feel magnificent about yourself, at long last realizing that you are in charge

3: you need sound nourishments to assist you with gauging your optimal weight

4: prepared presently to take the necessary steps to achieve this

5: eyes open, completely wakeful, splendid and alert, presently completely conscious. That right...

Weight Loss Psychology

Getting increasingly fit is on various occasions less troublesome if you are ordinarily sorted out it. This may sound fundamental, supposedly, most wellbeing food nuts quit their weight decrease plan not in light of the fact that they feel hungry or experience issues with the menus, however since of mental reasons. It is possible that, they become drained, or disappointed with their pace of weight decrease, or endure through a blasting oversight and become overwhelmed by fault or feel extravagantly "denied" proceeding. Likewise, starting there ahead, endeavoring to clarify their failure, a critical package of them charge their eating routine arrangement, their private condition or their innate slightness to get fit as a fiddle. This approach as frequently as potential rehashes itself. Along these lines, a few calorie counters can encounter years vainly attempting to shed pounds, while never understanding the genuine clarification behind their difficulty. Here are three shrouded mental issues we experience when endeavoring to shed pounds, close by unequivocal tips for how to smash them.

Issue 1. Not Knowing How Weight Loss Will Benefit You

Regardless of whether we need to lose 20 or 220 pounds, we need to change our dietary examples and maybe a few other lifestyle affinities also. Uncovering these improvements may not be irksome on Day 1 of Week 1 of our weight decrease diet, in light of the fact that our key excitement, when in doubt, gives us adequate inspiration. Normally inside 2-3 weeks, our "new" eating model begins to meddle with our standard lifestyle and, beside in case we are set up for this, our craving to keep eating less low-quality nourishment will start to darken. Rather than considering us to be as an overall ID to a transcendent weight and shape, we trust it to be a knot and a weight. It progresses toward ending up being something we are doing because we "must" as oppose to considering the way that we "have to." This is the primary huge, eager issue we experience while expending less calories.

To vanquish this issue, we need to know unquestionably why we are attempting to get increasingly fit. We need an undeniable thought of how it will benefit us. If we have an obvious preferred position to anticipate, will we have the decision to confine the drive to returned to our past antagonistic individual direct guidelines? General favorable circumstances from having a logically thin, lighter shape aren't adequately profound. We need a one-sided, unequivocal bit of leeway - something we can imagine - that organizes our idea. Possibly a shoreline occasion, or a fantasy outfit to wear for a particular event, or another shape to parade at Thanksgiving. Whatever we pick, it must make a disturbance inside our head! Keep in mind, the second we begin to feel that we "need to" accomplish something, it changes into the adversary - like settling regulatory duties or getting out the storm cellar - and our inspiration flies out the window. To accomplish enduring weight decrease, we need to "need it."

Issue 2. Trying to Be Perfect

During my 24 years or so as a weight decrease authority and nutritionist, I've met maybe 10,000 calorie counters eye to eye and look at in the end with another 100,000 over the Internet. In any case, so far, I haven't met one single gainful wellbeing food nut who was impeccable. Truth be told, the more important bit of my dynamic customers submitted immense proportions of bungles. They had unpleasant days, horrible weeks - even entire months - during which they went completely wild. In any case, none of this shielded them from winning at long last. Why not? Since they picked up from their mistakes. Moreover, we ought not disregard by a wide margin the majority of our self-information begins from the misunderstandings we make, not our triumphs.

Grievously, different wellbeing food nuts enthusiasm to attempt to be great. Along these lines, when they do tumble off the truck (as they generally do), they imagine that its difficult to drive forward through their "failure," and become overwhelmed by fault. So, notwithstanding the way that their pass may have been regularly irrelevant (a week's end gorge), they turn out harshly. Since, the accuse does authentic harm, not the pigging out.

The movement is this. When eating less carbs, don't relax around idly attempting to be perfect. It just prompts expanded fault and frustration. Or maybe, perceive that you will submit blunders, and don't permit them to divert you when they occur. Trust them to be a learning experience. For instance, in case you drink a huge amount of liquor when eating out, and enormously gorge, likewise, don't get up the following morning in an ambush of desolation. Or maybe, relish your experience, and welcome that you have made a fundamental exposure: that an over the top proportion of liquor makes weight decrease dynamically irksome. By responding thusly, you will keep up a key decent way from fault and imagine that its altogether simpler to come back to your eating routine.

Issue 3. With respect to Diet as Race

Another standard issue concerns the speed of weight decline. Different wellbeing food nuts might want to get increasingly fit exceptionally smart and are mentally wiped out arranged when their body doesn't carry on in this style. If seven days goes with no weight decline, they become disrupted and begin to lose interest. Shockingly, similar to it or not, the human body is proposed for perseverance, not "appearance." along these lines, it has no fervor for shedding muscle versus fat, which it sees as a basic wellspring of significance during times of starvation. Along these lines, the silliest extent of fat we can lose in seven days is around 3 pounds, while somebody who is under 30 pounds' overweight may lose around 1 pound. Anything extra is probably going to be a mix of water and muscle weight.

To pound your anxiety and keep enduring weight decrease, quit considering you're eating routine a race. Or maybe, trust it to be an endeavor. This decreases weight and gives you powerfully "breathing space" to sink into your new dietary examples. I clarify this in more detail on my unfathomable weight decrease discussion, and an impressive number of people imagine that it's an advantageous framework. Simultaneously, avoid bouncing on your bathroom scales each day - restrict yourself to once reliably. Checking your weight considerably more ordinarily requests that you take a transient perspective on things, which isn't useful.

I understand that "persisting" weight decrease may not sound unpleasantly captivating, apparently, the more moderate the weight decrease, the more it stays off. Moreover, as imparted above, in case you lose different pounds seven days, it won't be fat - it will be muscle or water. Likewise, recalling that losing water is basically passing - and along these lines silly - losing muscle will slow your retention and expansion the risk of future weight gain.

Thusly, when you start your next eating routine undertaking, recollect there's no flood. Set yourself a sensible weight decrease objective and let Nature finish to its genuine end. For instance, if you check 200 pounds and are going for 150 pounds, enable yourself a half year to appear at your goal. Moreover, in case it takes somewhat more, so what? At the edge of the day, what do you lose?

These three mental issues address incalculable eating routine dissatisfactions. Acing them will refresh your odds of shedding pounds. Along these lines, before you set out with all your standard vitality on one progressively "new" diet, set aside nearly a perfect chance to consider these issues totally and starting there forward, watch the pounds vanish.

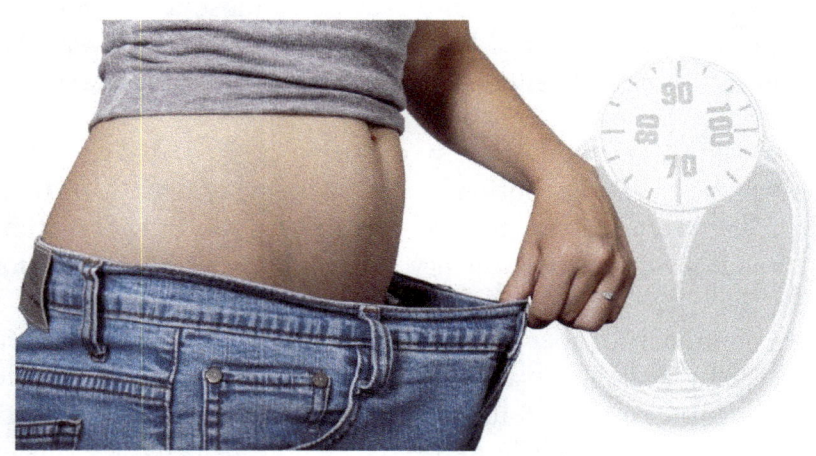

Affirmations for Weight Loss (Motivation)

1. I will partake in my wellbeing plan.
2. I am a decent sleeper. I rest adequately and wake up feeling rested.
3. I encircle myself with individuals who bolster my sound decisions.
4. I talk, think, and act in flawless wellbeing.
5. I decide to make every one of my considerations sound ones.
6. I love myself that is the reason I need to be solid.
7. My wellbeing is my most extreme need.
8. Being fit and sound falls into place without a hitch for me.
9. I am mindful that the best way to carry on with a satisfying life is to live a fun, sound and dynamic way of life.
10. I can without much of a stretch redirect myself from cafés and foundations that can fill in as a compulsion to rehearse undesirable dietary patterns.
11. I can without much of a stretch oppose prepared food, refined sugars, and salty bites.
12. I have built up another good dieting propensity.
13. I keep myself hydrated to help in my weight reduction.
14. I have set up a customary exercise routine that is simple for me to follow.
15. I have grasped an existence of spotless and sound living.
16. I have at long last arrived at my optimal weight.
17. I am fruitful in my objective of extraordinary weight reduction.
18. My body is light and adaptable and can without much of a stretch acclimate to all the new and sound changes.
19. My body is solid to bear the physical difficulties it is being exposed to.
20. My body is great, and I love myself by the day's end.
21. I can feel my body getting slimmer consistently.
22. I am a profoundly energetic individual and I have set my outrageous weight reduction objectives to something that I can accomplish and go past my desires.
23. I Believe in my ability to arrive at my objectives of outrageous weight reduction.

24. Every day I gauge myself, the scales show noteworthy weight reduction.

25. Each day I effectively get more fit as a matter of course.

26. My health improvement plan is working like enchantment.

27. I have an upbeat and sound disposition towards life.

28. I love my body that is the reason I need the best for it.

29. My body is reacting colossally to my weight reduction endeavors.

30. I can feel my body fats liquefying endlessly.

31. I have built up a high pace of digestion that encourages me arrive at my optimal weight.

32. I have total spotlight on my weight reduction venture.

33. When I set an objective, I ensure I accomplish it.

34. Every day I wake up tested and resolved to arrive at my optimal weight objective.

35. No one and nothing can restrain me from getting into the best state of my life.

36. My assurance to get more fit can't be deflected.

37. My inspiration to practice is outstanding.

38. Every day I am roused to follow an ordinary exercise routine.

39. I am self-roused and propelled to get in shape and follow a sound way of life.

40. Being solid isn't just a way of life for me however a rule that I am resolved to keep.

41. I decide to be a solid and fit individual.

42. I decide to eat soundly and keep up a functioning way of life.

43. I decide to feel fit and hot.

44. My psyche is hard-wired to need just solid food and my body consequently feels that requirement for every day physical movement.

45. My psyche just acknowledges Positive musings and praises about my body and opposes any negativities that can redirect me away from my weight reduction objective.

46. I am encircled by individuals who help and rouse me during my weight reduction venture.

47. I am deserving of acceptable wellbeing.

48. I spotlight on positive movement.

49. I am a companion to my body.

50. I take care of my body with unqualified sympathy.

51. It feels great to work out.

52. My digestion is working in my preferred position by helping me put on my ideal weight.

53. I am grateful for my body for all the things it accomplishes for me.

54. I comprehend what to eat and how to carry on with my life.

55. Every physical development I make causes me keep up my optimal body weight.

56. The more I move, the easier I feel.

57. My stomach is conditioned; my arms are conditioned I-am-fit as a fiddle.

58. I think that it's simple to remain fit as a fiddle.

59. I'm appreciative for my solid fit body.

60. I am in charge of how the measure of food I eat.

61. Following a smart dieting plan is simple for me.

62. Eating sound nourishments enables my body to get the entirety of the supplements it should be in the best shape.

63. My digestion is quick.

64. I recognize the excellence my body holds.

65. I have confidence in myself and recognize my enormity.

66. I bring the characteristics of adoration into my heart.

67. I can acknowledge myself for who I am.

68. Every day, I am drawing nearer to my optimal weight.

69. I am equipped for accomplishing my objectives.

70. I am upbeat about the sentiment of health these progressions are bringing me.

71. Every day, I progressively love my body.

72. Trusting my body is getting simpler.

73. I remain concentrated on my optimal size.

74. This is my body; I approach it with deference and respect.

75. I am content with my body.

76. My body is being reestablished to its normal condition of incredible wellbeing.

77. Love and friendship stream into my existence easily.

78. I acknowledge life.

79. All my most out of this world fantasies and each beneficial thing is streaming to me easily and without any problem.

80. I'm totally spurred to carrying on with a sound life.

81. I have the force in me to make beneficial things occur
82. I am turning out to be fitter and more grounded each day through exercise.
83. I commend my capacity to settle on great and solid decisions around food.
84. I eat well dinners.
85. Every day I am practicing and dealing with my body.
86. I am effectively controlling my weight through a mix of smart dieting and working out.
87. I keep up my optimal weight and I appreciate life being fit.
88. I love the inclination practicing gives me.
89. I discover time to work out.
90. When I work out, I feel ground-breaking and invigorated.
91. I am consuming calories consistently.
92. I love working out, I love working out, I love eating characteristic nourishments.
93. It is simple for me to control my weight.
94. I love the flavor of solid food.
95. It's energizing to find my remarkable food and exercise framework for my optimal weight.
96. Everything I eat mends feeds my body and encourages me arrive at my optimal weight.
97. I have a compelling impulse to eat just sound nourishments and to relinquish any prepared nourishments.
98. I just eat nutritious nourishments, and I can without much of a stretch oppose allurements.
99. I am so thankful since I have good dieting propensities.
100. Eating well falls into place without any issues for me.
101. Healthy nutritious food is the thing that I eat each day.
102. My body profits by the solid food that I eat.
103. Healing is going on in both my psyche and heart.
104. Healing occurs with each progression I take.
105. I effectively reach and keep up my optimal weight
106. I take the necessary steps to be sound.
107. Every day I am getting slimmer and more advantageous.
108. I am a delightful individual back to front.
109. I can genuinely cherish myself for who I am.

110. I am thankful for the body shape I have been honored with.

111. I acknowledge myself for who I am.

112. I am thankful for the body I have.

113. I am drawing nearer to my optimal load with every single day.

114. I am getting thinner since I need to and in light of the fact that I have the ability to do this.

115. Making changes is normal to me.

116. I am more beneficial and more grounded with every day that passes.

117. Today, I center around the beneficial things that are unfurling in my life.

118. Every day is a fresh start.

119. I love my excellent body.

120. I am content, tranquil and full filled.

121. I affectionately permit love, satisfaction and great wellbeing to move through my psyche and my body.

122. I am cherished and am adoring.

123. I am thankful forever and for my body.

124. I am serene, cheerful and focused.

125. I have faith in myself and I will succeed.

126. I frequently envision myself in my optimal weight

127. Exercising is fun, and it causes me to feel great.

128. I am joyfully practicing each day

129. I eat products of the soil day by day

130. Exercising is entertaining.

131. I am achieving and keeping up my ideal weight.

132. Every piece of my body is sound and fit.

133. I exercise, and I appreciate a solid, conditioned body.

134. Exercising works out easily for me.

135. I effectively deal with my weight through practicing and through smart dieting.

136. I work out and see the outcomes immediately in my vitality endurance and quality.

137. I'm turning out to be lighter and more grounded each day.

138. I consume calories effectively and as often as possible

139. I'm committing myself to remaining fit as a fiddle

140. I eat just when I am eager.

141. I eat nourishments that cause me to feel and look great.

142. I have a decent example of conduct around food.
143. My longing for fat-rich nourishments is dissolving.
144. My body digests food well and takes out the supplements I need.
145. I eat in appropriate segments.
146. Food is my fuel, so I give my body perfect, solid fuel.
147. My relationship with food is certain and solid.
148. I would already be able to see myself at my optimal weight.
149. I look and feel incredible.
150. I love my body.

Heal Your Relationship with Food

Too often we eat too much of what we need, and this can lead to unwanted weight gain.

Careful eating is important because it will help you appreciate food more. Instead of eating large portions to feel full, you will try each bite.

This will be easy for those who want to do it fast but need to do something to increase their will power by extending the periods between their hours. It will also be very useful for people who struggle with food. Controlling a portion alone may be enough for some people to see the natural results of their weight loss plan. Try your best to incorporate careful eating practices into your daily life so you can control how much you eat.

This meditation will be specific to eating an apple. You can practice careful eating without meditation, share your meals with others, or sit alone with a nice view out the window. This meditation will guide you to understand the types of thoughts that will be helpful while staying alert during meals.

Change your Mindset

The first step you must take on your weight loss journey is to change your mindset. This is the first and very important step to sustainable weight loss.

As you work to change your weight loss mindset, you are, in effect, rethinking what you really believe about losing weight, so that your overall weight loss journey serves you better.

In other words, you need to cultivate your own weight loss condition. This psychological change you must take can be even more difficult than adding a few additional herbs to your plate.

This is a thing that needs to be done. First of all, be aware that there are three words to keep in mind when embarking on this journey.

These words are "I can't", "I won't," and "I can't". These are three short words that you must ban to be successful, as they come from your mind and have virtually nothing to do with your inner strength or what you can achieve.

If you use them frequently, they can have a huge indirect effect on your weight loss journey and your level of fitness.

Therefore, you must reverse the entire scenario and leave the negative discussion behind. People trying to lose weight generally say so not just because of their past negative experiences.

For example, someone who says they don't like vegetables simply remembers old experiences that have nothing to do with their current behavior.

For this reason, their old experiences should not dictate their current behavior. If there are some that I can't or can't define in your vocabulary, you have to turn the script upside down and turn them into me and I can.

This will motivate and encourage you to go further and after several days you will be able to choose your new rhythm with ease.

If your current fitness level is low, the words "I can't" will hinder your success. Instead of saying I can't do ten push-ups, let's just say I'm trying to succeed. You have to try, as it is better to try and fail than fail.

You can start with two push-ups and with each new day add one more push to go further until you reach your fitness goal.

Your weight loss journey should start by changing your mindset and rewriting your thinking to lose weight

There are many natural ways to overcome your weight loss plateau, such as changing your eating habits and being physically active.

However, without changing your mindset, these tricks will only work in the short term by providing a sustainable weight loss journey, as there is always an underlying thought that keeps you away from sustainable weight loss.

If you don't go there and face it, you will continue fighting along the way.

For example, many women tend to lose weight as soon as they begin to make healthier dietary choices, but their weight loss progresses to a halt before they are completely satisfied with what they see in the mirror.

The truth is that losing weight sustainably is much more than losing those extra kilos that seem to melt at the beginning of the journey.

The trick is to keep losing weight after this initial period. Many women fail at this step because after periods of weight loss, their progress simply freezes.

The key reason for this to occur is that the very common weight loss plateau prevents you from losing weight in the long run.

To overcome this problem, there is no magic trick you can do other than change your weight loss mindset.

Overcome Your Weight Loss Plateau

The secret to overcoming your weight loss plateau is not in a secret diet plan or training program, but it is much deeper in your mind.

The first step you need to take to overcome your weight loss plateau is to identify the real reasons why you are overweight.

If you're overweight, the main reason is probably not a lack of exercise, but a lack of willpower or dietary choices.

Yes, these are all the factors that determine your weight and play an important role in your overall health, how your body looks and feels.

Though, these are only certain manifestation of the deeper, real reason behind your weight struggles.

For instance, those fat resources in the body work as some kind of body protection. When we accumulate fat, we, in fact, build a massive fat shield in order to protect the body from various kinds of threats.

Moreover, many of us struggle with different fears, many of us feel threatened all the time both subconsciously and consciously. In these cases, fat we accumulate may serve as a hiding point making us less visible and making us less noticeable, less shiny in the world.

Many individuals feel greatly disappointed in some areas of their lives, many of them feel as if they are not following any certain life purpose.

Some of them are also greatly unsatisfied with their personal relationships and they feel no real connection with friends and family members.

These people struggling with threats and disappointments tend to hide behind their body and tend to fill their inner void by turning to food.

The truth is that there are many other psychological reasons for your weight struggles other than your dieting choices and your lack of physical activity.

As you work on changing your mindset, it is extremely important that you also work on identifying those reasons.

It is important that you discover what is holding you back in order to get rid of those additional pounds for good.

Accept Current Reality

The next step requires that you truly accept your current reality. There are many females completely obsessing over their dieting plan, obsessing over counting calories, blaming their slow metabolism and wondering what went wrong.

This is extremely unhealthy bringing nothing good. In fact, thinking obsessively about weight loss, hating what you see in the mirror and thinking that your life would be much enjoyable if that excess fat were only a certain manifestation of the true thing which is keeping you from moving towards your goals.

Obsessing over these things, just shows that you are not accepting of your reality, that you resist it, and whatever you try to resist, it surely persists.

In order to overcome your weight loss plateau and in order to shed that stubborn excess weight, the first thing you are expected to do is to accept your current reality and work towards being okay with that.

This does not mean that you will stop your weight loss progress, but it means that by accepting your current reality, you can work towards a slimmer you in the future.

Once there, you will be completely free of those relative internal tensions which, once gone, make you more focused and motivated to keep reaching your goals.

Find Your Motivation

Many people, when thinking about the motivation for weight loss, what comes to mind is those media motivational weight loss posters with skinny models repeating washed out phrases we have heard many times before with no personal message.

These types of weight loss motivational posters are extremely superficial and, in many cases, even damaging.

Yes, they can motivate you for a short time period, but in the long run, this is not the kind of motivation you need to keep going.

Instead, you need to ask yourself what should be your own, your personal motivation without being conditioned by mass culture and media and their assumptions that being fit and skinny is what makes us happy and what makes our lives whole.

These assumptions in the majority of cases are not conscious at all and you should avoid them. Instead of resorting to mass culture and media, think about what is truly important to you, what your inner senses and connection are telling you.

Think about what you want to gain with your weight loss. Is it being full of energy or being completely confident in what you see in the mirror?

In pursuance of discovering your true weight loss motivation, you need to examine how you truly feel, you need to work on addressing your core values and finally take complete ownership over your life vision.

Your motivation must come from you as your unique, personal manifesto, not from some fitness magazine or workout poster you see.

Once you have identified your own weight loss motivation, you need to embrace your core value and let your own, personal vision in addition to your desired feelings, guide you towards reaching your goals.

This kind of motivation coming from within you is the only right motivation you need and once you have it, everything else will come naturally.

Portion Control Hypnosis

Whether you wish to shed many pounds or maintain a healthy weight, proper portion consumption is as necessary as the consumption of appropriate foods. The rate of obesity among youngsters and adults has increased partly owing to the increase in restaurant portions.

A portion is the total quantity of food that you eat in one sitting. A serving size is the suggested quantity of one particular food. For instance, the amount of steak you eat for dinner maybe a portion; however, three ounces of steak, maybe a serving. Controlling serving sizes helps with portion control.

Health Benefits of Portion Control

Serious health problems are caused by overeating. For example, type 2 diabetes, weight problems, high blood pressure, and many more. Therefore, when you are looking to lead a healthy lifestyle, portion control should be a significant priority.

Fullness and Weight Management

Feeling satiable, or having a sense of fullness, will affect the quantity you eat and the way you usually eat. According to the British Nutrition Foundation, eating smaller portions slowly increases the feeling of satiety after a meal.

Eating a little portion also allows your body to use the foods you eat right away for energy, rather than storing excess fat. Weight loss is not as simple as controlling portion size. However, once you learn to observe the amount of food you eat, you will begin to apply conscious eating, which can help you make healthier food choices.

When you eat too fast, you don't notice that your stomach is full. Eat slowly and listen to hunger tips to increase feelings of satiety and ultimately eat less food.

Improved digestion

Significantly larger serving sizes contribute to stomach upset and discomfort (caused by an enlarged stomach that presses on your other organs). Your gastrointestinal system works best when it is not full of food. Portion management can help you get rid of cramps and bloating after eating. Also, you may run the risk of catching fire, as having a full stomach will push hydrochloric acid back into your digestive system.

Save money

Eating smaller portions can generate monetary benefits, especially when eating out. In addition to consuming controlled portions, you don't need to buy as many groceries. Measuring portion percentages can make the cereal box and walnut package last longer than food right out of the container.

Take, for example, the method of applying portion management in restaurants: ordering children's meals, which are generally cheaper than adult meals and closer to the correct size to eat.

Adult portion sizes in restaurants will equal two, three, or even more servings. So, as soon as the food reaches your table, request an extraction container and remove half of the food from the plate. Take your food home and this way you will have two meals that are worth one.

How to Control the Portions Using Hypnosis?

Hypnosis can bring you into a state of deep relaxation and quickly train your mind to understand when to instinctively eliminate excess food and allow your digestion to be lighter and more comfortable. You can discover the pleasure of being in tune with what your body needs for food. Hypnosis will retrain your instincts to regulate the pins. While you relax and listen repeatedly to strong hypnotic phrases that will be absorbed by your mind. You may quickly begin to notice that:

Your mind is no longer frozen in food

Your abdomen and intestines feel lighter

Now you don't feel uncontrollable pins in times "out of food"

Of course, you forget to eat between meals

You start to enjoy a healthier lifestyle.

There is a somewhat simple self-hypnosis process to help you control your appetite and portions. In a shell, you are immersed in a psychological state and imagine a dial or a flip switch of some type that is symbolic of your craving and your real hunger. Then you repeatedly apply to develop a true sense of control, then you employ it out of the hypnotic state and when confronted with those things and circumstances to curb the perceived hunger and control your appetite.

Portion Control Hypnosis Exercise

Step 1: Get yourself into a comfortable position and one where you will remain undisturbed for the period of this exercise. Ascertain your feet are flat on the ground and hands not touching. Then once you are in position, calm yourself.

You can do that by using hypnosis tapes; they are basic processes to assist you in opening the door of your mind.

Step 2: You may prefer to deepen your hypnotic state. The best and most straightforward is imagining yourself in your favorite place and relaxing your body bit by bit. Keep focused on the session at hand (that is, watch out not to drift off) then go to the third step.

Step 3: Take a picture of a dial, a lever or a flippy switch of some kind that is on a box or mounted on a wall of some sort-let it fully control, your mind's eye. Notice the colors, the materials that it is created out of, and the way it indicates 0-10 to mark the variable degrees of your real hunger.

Notice wherever it is indicating currently let it show you how hungry you are. Remember when last you ate, what you ate, whether or not the hunger is genuine or merely reacting to a recent bout of gluttony and wanting to gratify that sensation!

Once you have established the dial, where it is set, and trusting that the reading is correct, then go to the subsequent step.

Step 4: Flip the dial down a peg and notice the effects taking place within you. Study your feedback and ascertain that it feels like you are moving your appetite with the dial. The more you believe you are affecting your appetite with the dial, the more practical its application in those real-life situations.

Practice turning it down even lower and start recognizing how you use your mind to change your perceived appetite utilizing a method that is healthy and helps keep you alert when you encounter circumstances with plenty of food supply. Tell yourself that the more you observe this, the better control you gain over your appetite.

You might even create a strong affirmation that accompanies this dial "I am in control of my eating" is one such straightforward statement. Word it as you wish and make sure it is one thing that resonates well with you.

Once you have repeated the meaningful affirmations to yourself severally with conviction, proceed to the next step.

Step 5: Visualize yourself during a future scenario, where there is going to be constant temptation to continue eating although you are full, or to consume an excessive amount. See the sights of that place, take a mental note of the other people there, notice the smells, hear the sounds. Become increasingly aware of how you are feeling in this place. Get the most definition and clarity possible then notice that once the temptation presents itself, you turn down the dial on your craving. You realize that you are not hungry to eat anymore, then repeat your positive affirmations to yourself a few more times to strengthen it.

Run through this future state of affairs severally on loop to make sure your mind is mentally rehearsed about your plan to respond.

Step 6: Twitch your little finger and toes, then open your eyes and proceed to observe your skills in real-life and spot how much control you have.

Portion Hypnosis Session

This hypnosis session will have a deeply relaxing effect on you, and that is why you shouldn't be listening to this while driving, operating machinery, or looking after anyone else. If you need to awaken for any reason, you will do so easily and become comfortably alert. It's also okay if you fall asleep. Your subconscious mind will continue to listen to my voice, and you will still benefit from this hypnosis session.

Hypnosis is very relaxing. It's safe and positive, and you are always completely and fully in control. Just trust in yourself, relax, and enjoy the experience.

So now, find a quiet and comfortable place, either sitting or lying down with your head supported. Find a place where you know you won't be disturbed, where you can remain for the duration of this hypnosis session, and we'll get started.

Now that you find yourself in a quiet and comfortable position, arms resting by your sides, legs uncrossed, let us begin to absorb ourselves in relaxation and calmness. This is a time to be as lazy as you want, to let yourself go, and to allow yourself to become deeply relaxed. So, begin relaxing now. Let the muscles soften. With the next exhalation, drop the shoulders, and allow the body to sink into the surface below. Beginning to let go of everything, all thoughts, all tensions, and tightness. Let go of everything and become deeply soothed, deeply calm, and deeply relaxed. Listening gently to the sound of my voice, any other sounds you may hear will fade into the distance. My voice will guide you with the deepest level of relaxation, including the mind and the body.

All you need to do is let go. Let go and follow the suggestions I make. All of the suggestions I make are here to benefit you. If your eyes are not already closed, do so gently now.

Take a long, slow, and steady breath in, all the way down into the stomach. Hold the breath for a moment and breathe out slow and steady. Focusing completely on the breath, letting go, and now relaxing a little more with each exhalation. Take another long, slow, and steady breath in all the way down to the bottom of the stomach. This time hold the breath for a moment longer, and breathing out, all the way out slowly and steadily, letting go of everything. Letting the shoulders drop a little as the muscles may go, softening any tension or tightness in the body. Take one slow and steady breath all the way down to the bottom of the stomach, holding the breath a moment longer again and breathing all the way out, feeling more centered, calmer, steadier, continuing to relax a little further and more deeply with every exhalation. While you're continuing with your deep, steady, relaxing, breathing, notice the eyelids. As you peek through the eyelids, what colors do you see reflecting back?

Is there a dominant color? Does the color move? Perhaps it swirls or flickers, or even takes certain shapes. Or does the color remain still? Stay with this for a moment. Hold the gaze. Become comfortable in the feeling, allow the feeling to soften and let it provide comfort. Let the comfort deepen, just focusing on the color. Gazing at the color, notice how the color creates a stillness within. Let any thoughts or interruptions move through the mind. Move through the mind, or even floating up and out of it. You are safe, you are special, you are calm, you are becoming even more calm with every slow and steady breath you take.

In a moment, I'm going to count down from five to one, and when I get to one, you will have relaxed all the way down to a deep and comfortable space.

5 - Deepen now that feeling of relaxation. Feeling a gentle warmth touching the skin, a calm and comfortable warmth that will spread down slowly from the top of the head to the tips of the toes. As that subtle sensation of warmth moves down through the body, every sound, every muscle that it touches, relaxes and unwinds. Beginning now at the top of the head, and feeling now as the relaxation spreads down, down through the scalp, across the forehead, the muscles of the forehead softening, flattening and letting go, you may even feel a gentle tingling in the scalp and forehead as the relaxation moves down and throughout. Letting that gentle warmth spread down the face, down over the eyes, down the sides of the face, and letting go. Feel the comfortable warmth and relaxation spreading, spreading farther down over the nose, the top lip, and now the bottom lip, down into the jaw, allowing the muscles in the jaw to soften, feeling it relaxing and letting go, more deeply relaxed. The whole head now feels relaxed, sinking farther down and drifting, floating.

4- As all the muscles in the head continue to relax even more, feel that gentle tingling, warmth and relaxation, moving down into the neck, through the back of the neck, the sides of the neck, and the front of the neck. Letting that relaxation spread down now, down into the shoulders, deep into the muscles of the shoulders, the fibers all letting go. Letting go just like an elastic band being released, moving into a relaxed and loose state. All tension and tightness decapitating. Your relaxation and calmness spreading down to the arms, through the biceps and triceps, to the elbows, the forearms, and down through the hands to the tips of the fingers. Allow the arms to let go simply. Let them sink more deeply down, noticing how they feel more relaxed and lighter. Noticing just how they feel with deep relaxation moving all the way down and through them.

3 - You can feel that calmness now, spreading down through the body. Now feeling that deep relaxation is ready to spread down all through the back. Beginning now, at the base of the neck, allowing relaxation to move slowly and deeply down through the back one vertebra at a time. Allowing the vertebrae to let go of any tension, feeling the whole of the back now, letting go. Letting go, and sinking down, down to the deepest level of relaxation, drifting and floating.

2 - Everything relaxing, everything feeling loose and heavy, feeling the calmness and comfort through the hips and thighs now moving down through the knees. Down, through the hips and shins. A relaxation spreading down through the foot, the sole of the foot, down into the toes. It is going down and down, drifting and floating more and more deeply relaxed.

1 - Everything feeling loose, heavy, light, relaxed. The whole body now feeling so relaxed, so heavily relaxed that even if you wanted to move an arm or leg it would take way too much energy to do so. You can enjoy this feeling of deep relaxation and letting go. You can enjoy it again, and again, and again, every time you listen to this deep relaxation. Every time you listen to my voice, and the words that I say, your body will instinctively follow the requests to relax, and it will relax more intently, more deeply each and every time. The more you relax, the more you can relax. Now that you are enjoying this peace and relaxation, your mind is interested and ready to welcome these positive and beneficial words that I say.

As you are relaxing, now, take a moment to congratulate yourself on this wonderful journey that you're on. Give yourself a pat on the back because you're doing great. You're doing great because you've taken the first step. You've already taken the step to start. You've started, which is well beyond the point where many people have stopped. It's hard to believe, isn't it? However, many people don't get this far, unfortunately for them. These people won't ever see a positive change in themselves. Nothing is going to change when they keep on doing the same old things. You know that because you're different, and because you're different, you're already changing. You're doing a mind-shift, and a physical shift is about to come. You've managed to move forward. You're empowering yourself right now, just by getting started. You're listening to this progressive hypnosis program, and you do know that now that you've started, there's no turning back.

You're not a quitter.

You're in this for the long haul.

You want this.

You really want this.

You're ready and committed, and this is your time, your health, and your pride.

So, it's important to know why you want this, and I mean really know. What's your reason for wanting to become slimmer? Do you want to become healthier? Do you need to improve your health? Will being slimmer improve your posture, remove aches and pains? Do you want to be around longer for the sake of your family? Do you have special people in your life who can't afford to lose you? Do you want to walk into a clothing store and buy them off the rack? Do you want to return to a previous smaller size?

Do you want to wear clothes that increase your confidence and imitate your style instead of bigger and baggy clothes?

What is the most important reason to you for becoming slimmer? The answer will come to you instantly. Lock it in now.

Self-Hypnosis Session to Stop Sugar Cravings

Sometimes when we are on the journey of weight loss, we might find that we are continually monitoring our cravings and attempting to avoid overindulging in the foods that are not healthy for us. We might find ourselves wanting to indulge in foods that are not in alignment with our diet or wanting to indulge in foods that we know have gotten us in this situation, to begin with. Sometimes the cravings are so difficult that we forget that we have a choice of whether or not we are going to eat these foods.

This fifteen-minute meditation will help you remember that you have a choice and will help you make the right choice to help keep you on track with your weight loss journey.

Start by sitting in a comfy spot...

Let yourself relax into a comfortable position as you feel yourself being supported by the chair you have chosen to sit on...

Rest your hands over your abdomen so that you can feel your stomach rise and fall with each breath...

Notice how easily the breath comes in and out...

Notice how comfortable it is to let the breath flow naturally through your body...

When you are ready, take a deep breath in through your nose...

And then let it out through your mouth...

Again, take a deep breath in through your nose...

And out through your mouth...

One more time, feel the breath coming in through your nose and filling your lungs up with rich oxygen...

And then exhale through your mouth, feeling all of the air completely exit your body... Then let your breath return to its natural rhythm...

Now, when you are completely relaxed, I want you to imagine a room that has a table and a chair at it...

I want you to walk towards that chair slowly, one step at a time...

When you reach it, I want you to pull the chair out and sit down in it...

Notice how comfortable it is...

Notice how fully it supports you, and how it seems as though the chair was perfectly made for you...

And in front of you on the table, notice a placemat with an empty plate on top of it...

On the table in front of you, I want you to imagine several dishes of food...

About half is filled with the foods you are craving and would love to eat right now...

And the other half is filled with delicious, healthy foods that you are struggling to fall in love with...

I want you to fill your plate up with the foods you are craving...

Anything you are craving that you know you shouldn't be eating right now...

I want you to fill your plate up... Take more than you need... And then sit down in your chair and look at the plate filled with all of your favorite foods...

Now, I want you to imagine a garbage can next to the table...

And I want you to picture yourself standing up and walking over to that garbage can, with your plate in your hands...

I want you to then dump most of the food off of your plate, leaving only a few bites of each type of food on the plate...

Then, I want you to return to your place setting, and put your plate back on the table...

When you are ready, start spooning the helpings of the other dishes onto your plate...

Notice the rich colors...

Inhale the unique aromas with each dish...

Imagine the way your body will be nourished and fulfilled by the nutrition in each dish...

Once your plate is full, I want you to look at your plate...

Now is where you get to decide...

You get to decide where you want to start on that plate...

You get to decide what you want to eat first, and what you want to eat last...

Because you see, you have the total authority to decide what foods you do and don't want to indulge in...

No matter what cravings you may or may not be having...

You can decide to overindulge...

Or to enjoy a few bites and then resume eating your healthy diet...

You see, losing weight is not a matter of depriving yourself of what you love, unless you choose to...

Losing weight is about changing your lifestyle to foster a healthier diet... And healthier habits...

That will support your body and nourish you with rich vitamins and minerals...

And if you choose...

You can enjoy a few bites of what you crave...

Because you are the one who gets to decide...

And should you decide you don't want any bites at all...

Well, that is your decision too...

Because you are the only one who gets to decide what goes into your body...

Not your cravings...

Not your habits... Not the contents of your fridge... Not the influence of your friends or family... You...

You are the one who decides what you will eat... And what you won't eat...

So, whether you choose to enjoy those few bites of the food you crave... Or whether you choose to put them in the trash with the rest of it...

That is completely up to you...

When you are ready, I want you to return your awareness to the room...

And when you awaken completely from your meditative state... I want you to remember that you are in charge of what you eat... No one else... Only you...

And you have the power to choose wiser, healthier decisions.

Eliminate cravings

Imagine a scenario in which you could disconnect from your desires. Seclude them and send them away? Some weight reduction hypnotic systems assist you with doing this. For instance, you may be approached to imagine sending your yearnings – state on a ship ceaselessly out to the ocean. Recommendations can likewise help you reframe your yearnings and figure out how to oversee them all the more adequately.

It can be tempting to give into the promises we see from celebrities and other big brand ads about losing weight. They make it seem so effortless and fun, but when we start the journey ourselves, we soon discover that it is not so easy. This hypnosis is a process that will aide in your weight loss journey and provide for you a natural way to shed the pounds.

You will be guided through the process of feeling better, mindful eating, goal-oriented thoughts, and dedication to the body. This hypnosis is a little different than others and will involve "I" statements. Allow these thoughts to come into your brain as if they were your own.

Causes of Emotional Eating

The vast majority had eaten at once or another for enthusiastic reasons. When there's the strain, it very well may be the go-to feeling. I review a few times when one individual would state to associates, "I'm ravenous who needs to get something with me (which means something sweet)?" We were totally depleted and realized only eating.

Gobbling to control feelings can wind up having some negative impacts over an extensive stretch of time. One of the principle issues with utilizing food to control feelings is that it can prompt weight issues, and much more issues accompany weight.

Eating for passionate reasons for existing is utilized to calm any of an assortment of feelings like discouragement, rage, disillusionment, forlornness or fatigue, to give some examples. Passionate appetite isn't equivalent to physical yearning (the genuine explanation behind eating), and you're searching for food to address intense subject matters. We realize that food cannot really satisfy an enthusiastic need, as it is planned to ease physical yearning.

The beginning stage for passionate eating is to learn in case you're engaging in it. Verily, numerous individuals are uninformed of what they are doing, accepting that they are really indulging. The nourishments picked for enthusiastic eating will in general be the ones you would discover comfort nourishments: high in fat, salt and sugar. Here are some enthusiastic eating signs:

• You eat when you're not ravenous.
• Eat when you have an inclination that you are.
• Eat peacefully.
• Eating a short time later and feeling regretful.
• Eating to an extreme, and not knowing why.
• Eating to keep yourself feeling much improved.
• For no clear explanation, longing for a bite, and feeling you can't survive without it.

Enthusiastic eating can be invigorating on the grounds that, from the outset, it tastes great, and there are altogether the idealistic emotions about the amount you need or need it. The nice sentiments (help, quiet) from enthusiastic eating will just keep going for a specific measure of time (one moment to hours) trailed by a defining moment where you experience the accompanying circumstances:

• Appointed liable.
• Feeling embarrassed.
• Feeling aggravated that you are exaggerating yourself.
• Feeling a recovery of the underlying sensation causing the gorge.
• Feel furious that you've shed pounds or perhaps put on weight.

The last final product is that enthusiastic eating doesn't work to mitigate the underlying feeling that sent you to the food. Understanding this is the beginning stage for this conduct to move. Save it for yourself. Frequently praise yourself that no doubt about it now. You can want to beat yourself to do as such for a really long time. This reasoning cycle doesn't help you in any productive manner, be that as it may, yet rather take you back to gorging in light of the fact that you are frantic at yourself for indulging (a round cycle).

Stop Emotional Eating Hypnosis

A few of us have partaken in passionate eating for sooner or later. Enthusiastic eating happens in the event that we eat to mitigate injured sentiments or adapt to an unpleasant circumstance. Passionate eating can happen in the wake of a difficult day at work, a battle with a friend or family member, or when the children go around the house crying. The initial step to maintaining a strategic distance from passionate eating is to become cognizant that it is happening. Over the span of the day, ask yourself ordinarily how you feel to stop a lot of strain. Perceive the indications of distress or strain. Figure out how to pass on the sentiments productively so they can be distributed. Holding in negative or destructive sentiments may prompt a gorge later on. Halting to assess your feelings during the day can likewise assist you with delaying before going after unfortunate nourishments.

Second, forestalling causes. Recall the last enthusiastic eating second. What happened not long before you'd eat? Recollect not being ravenous and taking care of at any rate? Do you despite everything eat after a troublesome activity meeting or contest with an associate? Recognizing and forestalling enthusiastic eating exercises can help dissuade potential events.

Third, take a stab at accomplishing something different while eating occurs. By checking your passionate state during the day, you will be aware of when enthusiastic eating will happen and looking for answers for it. When eating swelling nourishments causes you to feel sure and loose, form a rundown of different propensities adding to similar emotions. Exercise is a significant method to advance positive emotions. Different proposals like hot showers, perusing a decent book or viewing your preferred film.

Eat Healthy with Subliminal Hypnosis

You will go through a little while or longer cautiously watching the sorts of nourishment you eat and your dietary patterns, by and large, going from nourishment planning to calories per feast, the carb admission and protein levels, yet you're experiencing episodes of misery and go to reflection, not a drug to work out of burdensome States of the psyche when they happen, and frequently your weight gain is credited to melancholy.

When something unpleasant will happen, or emotion of dejection or an episode of self-uncertainty will catch a day, and you will hope to comfort in foods you ought not to eat. You know not to purchase that case of treats, yet you do in any case and devour the crate with a gallon of milk, for instance. Or on the other hand, rather than the natural product, you will arrange French fries imagining that only one time won't damage and afterward end up doing likewise once more.

Like a pendulum, you influence to and from among slimming down and enjoying your preferred solace foods, moving to start with one outrageous then onto the next. First, you observe each calorie you expend; next, you end up heading the other way, capitulating to the impulse to enjoy comfort foods. Eating fewer carbs causes you to need comfort foods even more, and after you have suppressed your craving for them, it breaks out even more energetically. This is the point at which you begin requesting French fries rather than organic products once more.

Wretchedness prompts indulging, while bliss permits you to consume fewer calories. So, in the last investigation, both despondency and happiness are defining moments as you influence starting with one extraordinary then onto the next - clearly sadness can't be just thing that changes your dietary patterns.

Actually, extraordinary eating fewer carbs is the thing that makes you out of nowhere want French fries. So, what would it be a good idea for you to do? Eat French fries constantly? Certainly not. Since this is the other outrageous that will toss you directly once more into consuming less calories mode.

Each activity has an equivalent and inverse response, so forcing anything excessively inflexible on your body can't remain without outcomes. In the event that you yield to the impulse to slim down, you will incite new episodes of gorging, prompting new episodes of despondency.

What you have to do is drop both indulging and slimming down without a moment's delay. Except if you shut down the two limits, you will end up influencing to and fro between them until the end of time.

How to Use Hypnosis to Change Eating Habits?

1. Think yourself thin and implement affirmations to help you get there in a healthy and sustainable way by adopting the habits of people who have already reached their weight and body positivity goals.

2. Adjust your mind to assist your weight loss goals and support it every day.

3. Don't eat without thinking, which includes both emotional eating, binge eating, and any act of mindless eating. Recognize the differences between emotional eating and eating because you are hungry.

4. Enjoy cooking and fill your home with good food instead of anything tempting. This will also help you to develop more controlled eating patterns. By not filling your home with sugary or fatty foods, you're instantly making a change. Although it's difficult, it's a bold one to be proud of.

5. Don't eat because of comfort; that usually leads to the over-consumption of calories.

6. Don't be reckless. If you're going to spend almost all your time sitting in front of a television binge-watching your favorite series, you're bound to want to snack. Stay true to your affirmations and believes during hypnosis and remind yourself to stay active throughout the day. This will prevent eating out of boredom and potentially lead to more weight-loss.

7. Stay motivated throughout your journey with hypnosis. Remembering that you're not going to achieve results overnight, but in the long haul, it is the answer to keeping both your mind and body in check.

stop sugar cravings hypnosis

Is it forbidden in this world to leave out sugar (as much as possible) in your diet? I'm talking about white sugar or brown sugar or added sugar, and not about natural sugars that you find in fruit or honey for example. Is it forbidden?

I ask because as soon as a person gives up on sugar there can be a big hoo-hah about the whole thing. When you say 'no' to a slice of cake or a dessert, for example, some will stop and try to advise you and tell you that moderation is key. It's as if you are doing something wrong. But what's wrong with having had enough of something. Enough is enough. You can make cakes and desserts which are very sweet and tasty which have no sugar in them except for natural sugars and enjoy life much more compared to before with new and higher levels of energy and without feeling as if you're missing out on anything. So, what's the fuss? Ok, sometimes some individuals will actually get jealous and try to sabotage your new positive resolution for their own evil kicks. But live and let live. If that's what makes them happy (impossible, it actually makes them more miserable) then so be it.

I have finally taken sugar out of my life.

Some time ago I remember people telling me that I had put on weight and often used to comment on my protruding stomach. I didn't mind for years. I always had a brief belief that if I wanted, I could get rid of it with some sit-ups. But this time I found myself standing outdoors one evening in the moonlight and looking down at my stomach. There it was. A piece of work. The result of all the chocolate, cakes, junk food, soft drinks, desserts, and sweets. It didn't feel too good either. I often felt bloated and I often felt so much discomfort that I often suspected that there might be something wrong with my insides.

I made a firm resolution and intention to get rid of the stomach once and for all.

I looked into how to get rid of stomach fat and found out what everyone besides myself already knew, sugar turns to fat.

The next day I stopped eating chocolate, cakes, sweets or anything with sugar in it. I stopped using sugar to my tea and coffee and either had them plain or with a bit of honey. Some tried to say that honey also has sugar, but I explained that this was natural and beneficial sugars and the same with fruits.

Instead of sugary soft drinks, I went for Apple juice. It has been well over 4 months now and even though I have not been working out as much as I intended, I have still lost weight and my stomach is shrinking.

Sugar turns to fat and sugar is very bad for your overall health. We are not talking about natural sugars and fruit sugars. No. We are talking here of unhealthy added sugar.

For the first several weeks shopping became interesting. All of a sudden, I was restricted in what I could buy because I realized that most of the food in the supermarkets contained added sugar.

I used to have cakes, sweets, desserts, and chocolate at night but now I have fruit, date, dried fruits, crisps or nuts, tea or coffee with or without honey. It's so easy. Not once did I suffer any difficulty or withdrawal as I am free to have fruit and honey if I fancy something sweet.

I remember how I used to wish I could eat more dates as they are so beneficial but used to find them too sweet. This was because I already had plenty of unnatural refined sugar in my diet that I couldn't stomach any sweeter things like real fruit or dried fruit.

However, to my surprise after around a week of not adding sugar to my tea and coffee, not having any chocolate, cakes, desserts, soft drinks or sweets, I found myself gobbling up apples, oranges, DATES, and dried fruit! It was like I needed a fix and I had to have the natural sugars that these foods contain.

This didn't last that long however and today I simply habitually have these things every day but not as much as before without even thinking about it.

The craving for sweet things like dates and fruit only lasted 2 weeks at the most. Now I add a tiny bit of honey to my tea or coffee whenever I can, or I just have it without.

Step by Step Instructions to Overcome Junk Food Cravings with Weight Loss Hypnosis

1."Reset" Your Fast Food Attachment

Weight reduction hypnotherapy is probably the simplest approaches to improve your outlook towards undesirable food without encountering inordinate yearnings or sentiments of insufficiency.

For a great many people, expending inexpensive food is either an imprudent choice or a passionate one. They have to exercise will to stop the energy, and this procedure will commonly prompt an inclination that they are looted or restricted.

You will modify the reaction instrument through spellbinding. Great practices are fun, and the conduct improves. You figure out how to adapt well, which implies you don't need to depend on nourishment for comfort any longer. Resetting the association liberates your brain and body with the goal that you have a ton of fun during the procedure of weight reduction.

2. Get Motivated

The correct motivation will help you in moving mountains. You must have the correct reasons on the off chance that you need to dispose of inexpensive food until the end of time.

A great many people don't understand that eating nutritious nourishments benefits their physical prosperity much more than appearance. By mesmerizing of weight reduction, individuals recognize what great consolation is and what significant job it plays during the time spent weight reduction.

Achievement infers valuable support. You need not keep yourself to finding the universe of adjusted eating. You will discover it unbelievably non-horrendous and even agreeable on the off chance that you are energetic about the change.

3. Connect with Your Emotions

the time or think that it's hard to manage worry in some other manner. Reaching internal emotions and uncertain issues will have the force and inspiration never to feel the requirement for inexpensive food.

Have you considered a habitual overeater? Is it accurate to say that you were viewed as a cheap food addict by others? Assuming this is the case, you despite everything have psychological weight to manage.

hypnosis will permit you to interface with these internal sentiments. You will comprehend why you're apprehensive, desolate, discouraged, or negative. Correspondence and realizing these negative sentiments can facilitate the way toward looking for an answer without slipping into shoddy nourishment for comfort.

And because you have some inadequate nourishments in your home toss it hard and fast. Try not to leave anything in your home that can prompt enticement.

And because you have companions who don't comprehend or bolster your excursion, put your association with them on delay. Mercifully reveal to them that you will connect again when all is good and well.

You are not sufficient (yet) to not surrender to enticements so you have to evacuate them just for the time being. When you are sufficient then you can return to it.

Lousy nourishment can be quite addictive. That is one of the main logics why such a significant number of individuals cannot change their dietary propensities. You need productive support and a sensible objective to achieve the change. A trance inducer will assist you with getting clear and pick the system which prompts enthusiastic and physical change.

Mindful Eating Benefits

The upsides of eating mindfully are unimaginable and realizing these points of interest is fundamental as you think about the activity.
• When you're anxious, you figure out how to eat and stop when you're plunking down.
• You figure out how to taste nourishment and acknowledge great sustenance tastes.
• You start to see gradually that unfortunate nourishment isn't as scrumptious as you accepted, nor does it make you feel extremely pleasant.
• Because of the over three points, if you are overweight, you will regularly get more fit.
• You start arranging your nourishment and eating through the passionate issues you have. It requires somewhat more, yet it's basic.
• Social overeating can turn out to be less of an issue—you can eat mindfully while mingling, rehearsing, and not over-alimenting.
• You begin to appreciate the experience of eating more, and as an outcome, you will acknowledge life more when you are progressively present.
• It can transform into a custom of mindfulness that you anticipate.
• You learn for the day how nourishment impacts your disposition and vitality.
• You realize what fuel your training best with nourishment, and you work and play.
A Guide to Mindful Eating
Keeping up a contemporary, quick-paced way of life can leave a brief period to oblige your necessities. You are moving always starting with one thing then onto the next, not focusing on what your psyche or body truly needs. Rehearsing mindfulness can help you to comprehend those necessities.
When eating mindfulness is connected, it can help you recognize your examples and practices while simultaneously standing out to appetite and completion related to body signs.
Originating from the act of pressure decrease dependent on mindfulness, rehearsing mindfulness while eating can help you focus on

74

the present minute instead of proceeding with ongoing and unacceptable propensities.

Careful eating is an approach to begin an internal looking course to help you become increasingly aware of your nourishment association and utilize that information to eat with joy.

The body conveys a great deal of information and information, so you can start settling on cognizant choices as opposed to falling into programmed — and regularly feeling driven — practices when you apply attention to the eating knowledge. You are better prepared to change your conduct once you become aware of these propensities.

Individuals that need to be cautious about sustenance and nourishment are asked to:

• Explore their inward knowledge about sustenance—different preferences

• Choose sustenance that please and support their bodies

• Accept explicit sustenance inclinations without judgment or self-analysis

• Practice familiarity with the indications of their bodies beginning to eat and quit eating.

General Principles of Mindful Eating

One methodology to careful eating depends on the core values given by Rebecca J. Frey, Ph.D., and Laura Jean Cataldo, RN: tune in to the internal craving and satiety signs of your body Identify private triggers for careless eating, for example, social weights, amazing sentiments, and explicit nourishments.

Here are a few tips for getting you started.

- Start with one meal. It requires some investment to begin with any new propensity. It very well may not be simple to make cautious eating rehearses constantly. However, you can practice with one dinner or even a segment of a supper. Attempt to focus on appetite sign and sustenance choices before you start eating or sinking into the feelings of satiety toward the part of the arrangement—these are phenomenal approaches to begin a routine with regards to consideration.

- Remove view distractions place or turn off your phone in another space. Mood killers such the TV and PC and set away whatever else —, for example, books, magazines, and papers—that can divert you from eating. Give the feast before your complete consideration.

- Tune in your perspective when you start this activity, become aware of your attitude. Perceive that there is no right or off base method for eating, yet simply unmistakable degrees of eating background awareness. Focus your consideration on eating sensations. When you understand that your brain has meandered, take it delicately back to the eating knowledge.
- Draw in your senses with this activity. There are numerous approaches to explore. Attempt to investigate one nourishment thing utilizing every one of your faculties. When you put sustenance in your mouth, see the scents, surfaces, hues, and flavors. Attempt to see how the sustenance changes as you cautiously bite each nibble.
- Take as much time as necessary. Eating cautiously includes backing off, enabling your stomach related hormones to tell your mind that you are finished before eating excessively. It's a fabulous method to hinder your fork between chomps. Additionally, you will be better arranged to value your supper experience, especially in case you're with friends and family.

Rehearsing mindfulness in a bustling globe can be trying now and again; however, by knowing and applying these essential core values and techniques, you can discover approaches to settle your body all the more promptly. When you figure out how much your association with nourishment can adjust to improve things, you will be charmingly astounded — and this can importantly affect your general prosperity and wellbeing.

Formal dinners, be that as it may, will, in general, assume a lower priority about occupied ways of life for generally people. Rather, supper times are an opportunity to endeavor to do each million stuff in turn. Consider having meals at your work area or accepting your Instagram fix over breakfast to control through a task.

The issue with this is you are bound to be genuinely determined in your decisions about healthy eating and eat excessively on the off chance that you don't focus on the nourishment you devour or the way you eat it.

That is the place mindfulness goes in. You can apply similar plans to a yoga practice straight on your lunch plate". Cautious eating can enable you to tune in to the body's information of what, when, why, and the amount to eat," says Lynn Rossy, Ph.D., essayist of The Mindfulness-Based Eating Solution and the Center for Mindful Eating director. "Rather than relying upon another person (or an eating routine) to reveal to you how to eat, developing a minding association with your own body can achieve tremendous learning and change."

From the ranch to the fork — can help you conquer enthusiastic eating, make better nourishment choices, and even experience your suppers in a crisp and ideally better way. To make your next dinner mindful, pursue these measures.

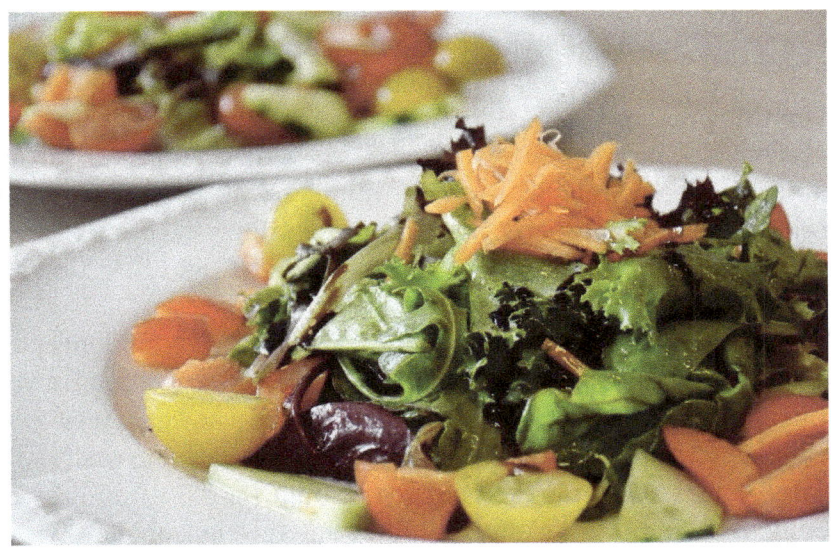

The Golden Method of Burning Fat Quickly and Permanently Through Hypnosis

Since we've already debunked the conspiracy theories on whether hypnosis is a form of mind-control practiced by individuals with hidden agendas, let's dive right into all of the hype that surrounds the idea of its effectivity.

Hypnosis plays an important role in medicinal solutions. In modern-day society, it is recommended for treating many different conditions, including obesity or weight loss in individuals who are overweight. It also serves patients who have undergone surgery extremely well, particularly if they are restricted from exercising after surgery. Given that it is the perfect option for losing weight, it is additionally helpful to anyone who is disabled or recuperating from an injury.

Once you understand the practice and how it is conducted, you will find that everything makes sense. Hypnosis works for weight loss because of the relationship between our minds and bodies. Without proper communication being relayed from our minds to our bodies, we would not be able to function properly. Since hypnosis allows the brain to adopt new ideas and habits, it can help push anyone in the right direction and could potentially improve our quality of living.

Adopting new habits can help eliminate fear, improve confidence, and inspire you to maintain persistence and a sense of motivation on your weight loss journey. Since two of the biggest issue's society faces today are media-based influences and a lack of motivation, you can easily solve any related issues by simply correcting your mind.

Correcting your mind is an entirely different mission on its own, or without hypnosis, that is. It is a challenge that most get frustrated with. Nobody wants to deal with themselves. Although that may be true, perhaps one of the best lessons hypnosis teaches you is the significance of spending time focusing on your intentions. Practicing hypnosis daily includes focusing on certain ideas. Once these ideas are normalized in your daily routine and life, you will find it easier to cope with struggles and ultimately break bad habits, which is the ultimate goal.

In reality, it takes 21 consecutive days to break a bad habit but only if a person remains persistent, integrating both a conscious and consistent effort to quit or rectify a habit. It takes the same quantity of time to adopt a new healthy habit. With hypnosis, it can take up to three months to either break a bad habit or form a new one. However, even though hypnosis takes longer, it tends to work far more effectively than just forcing yourself to do something you don't want to do.

Our brains are powerful operating systems that can be fooled under the right circumstances. Hypnosis has been proven to be genuine for breaking habits and adopting new ones due to its powerful effect on the mind. It can be measured in the same line of consistency and power as affirmations. Now, many would argue that hypnosis is unnecessary and that completing a 90-day practice of hypnotherapy to change habits for weight loss is a complete waste of time. However, when you think about someone who needs to lose weight but can't seem to do it, then you might start reconsidering it as a helpful solution to the problem. It's no secret that the human brain requires far more than a little push or single affirmation to thrive. Looking at motivational video clips and reading quotes daily is great, but is it really helping you to move further than from A to B?

It's true that today, we are faced with a sense of rushing through life. Asking an obese or unhealthy individual why they gained weight, there's a certainty that you'll receive similar answers.

Could it be that no one has time to, for instance, cook or prep healthy meals, visit the gym or simply move their bodies? Apart from making up excuses as to why you can't do something, there's actual evidence hidden in the reasons why we sell ourselves short and opt for the easy way out.

Could it be that the majority of individuals have just become lazy?

Regardless of your excuses, reasons or inabilities, hypnosis debunks the idea that you have to go all out to get healthier. Losing weight to improve your physical appearance has always been a challenge, and although there is no easy way out, daily persistence and 10 to 60 minutes a day of practice could help you to lose weight. Not just that, but it can also restructure your brain and help you to develop better habits, which will guide you in experiencing a much more positive and sustainable means of living.

Regardless of the practice or routine you follow at the end of the day; the principle of losing weight always remains the same. You have to follow a balanced diet in proportion with a sustainable exercise routine.

By not doing so is where most people tend to go wrong with their weight loss journeys. It doesn't matter whether it's a diet supplement, weight loss tea, or even hypnosis. Your diet and exercise routine still play an increasingly important role in losing weight and will be the number one factor that will help you to obtain permanent results. There's a lot of truth in the advice given that there aren't any quick fixes to help you lose weight faster than what's recommended. Usually, anything that promotes standard weight loss, which is generally about two to five pounds a week, depending on your current Body Mass Index (BMI), works no matter what it is. The trick to losing weight doesn't necessarily lie in what you do, but rather in how you do it.

When people start with hypnosis, they may be very likely to quit after a few days or weeks, as it may not seem useful or it isn't leading to any noticeable results.

Nevertheless, if you remain consistent with it, eat a balanced diet instead of crash dieting, and follow a simple exercise routine, then you will find that it has a lot more to offer you than just weight loss. Even though weight loss is the goal of this guidebook, it's important to keep in mind that lasting results don't occur overnight. There are no quick fixes, especially with hypnosis.

Adopting the practice, you will discover many benefits, yet two of the most important ones are healing and learning how to activate the fat burning process inside of your body.

Fat Burning Activation with Hypnosis

Hypnosis is not a diet, nor is it a fast-track method to get you where you want to go. Instead, it is a tool used to help individuals reach their goals by implementing proper habits. These habits can help you achieve results by focusing on proper diet and exercise. Since most weight-related issues are influenced by psychological issues, hypnosis acts as the perfect tool, laying a foundation for a healthy mind.

Hypnosis is not a type of mind control, yet it is designed to alter your mind by shifting your feelings toward liking something that you might have hated before, such as exercise or eating a balanced diet. The same goes for quitting sugar or binge eating. Hypnosis identifies the root of

80

the issues you may be dealing with and works by rectifying it accordingly. Given that it changes your thought pattern, you may also experience a much calmer and relaxed approach to everything you do.

Hypnosis works by maintaining changes made in the mind because of neuroplasticity. Consistent hypnotherapy sessions create new patterns in the brain that result in the creation of new habits. Since consistency is the number one key to losing weight, it acts as a solution to overcome barriers in your mind, which is something the majority of individuals struggle with. Hypnosis can also provide you with many techniques to meet different goals, such as gastric band hypnosis, which works by limiting eating habits, causing you to refrain from overeating.

Step by Step Hypnotherapy for Weight Loss

If you want to lose weight, you can rely on countless diets and exercise, but in recent years you can also rely on more innovative things. Let's take a look at a step-by-step guide that explains how to use hypnosis to lose weight.

Hypnosis therapy for weight loss can be used in a way that helps control hunger and nervous cravings, especially those caused by stress and the fact that you are eating at the same time. It is time to notice how this works, how many sessions should be done, and that it is not effective.

Steps to lose weight using hypnosis

- Hypnosis for weight loss is an effective treatment to reduce urges and desires and leave food vices, but the first thing to know is that it is `` help " and it can It is not a replacement.
- However, research has shown that some people have lost more than twice their weight because of hypnosis compared to those who did without treatment. Not only that, they improved their eating habits and improved their body image. On the other hand, a meta-analysis conducted by British researchers found that hypnosis can help regulate the release of peptides that control hunger and satiety mechanisms.
- Therefore, hypnosis is usually aimed at nervous, emotional people, as well as those who eat at night. Very often we eat due to lack of willpower and compensation (maybe we feel lonely, stressed and depressed, food seems to give us temporary relief). The goal of hypnosis is to break this wrong link.

- This treatment does not use a pendulum that swings in front of the nose to close the eyes. The patient and the hypnotherapist will have a conversation (about 25 minutes) during the hypnosis about what the patient's goal is, what is the trigger for hunger, and what diet will be followed.

In addition, experts suggest ways to deal with crisis moments when patients rely on food. Personalized therapist advice because there are different stories for each individual.

Hypnotherapy for Food Addiction

The national occasions start and with it the enticements of delectable choripanes, broils, empanadas, seismic tremors and a large group of different nourishments, a circumstance that turns into a genuine test for the person who experience the ill effects of issues to control their weight and dietary problems.

A couple of days before the national occasions start, there are a few who are as of now getting ready to appreciate a few days of festivities, a circumstance that turns into a genuine test for the individuals who have issues controlling their weight. Empanadas, choripanes, anticuchos and tremors are the allurements and genuine foes of the individuals who experience the ill effects of dietary problems or genuine food fixation.

In any case, fortunately, as other wild wants, hunger can likewise be controlled through mental treatments or hypnotherapies with extraordinary adequacy, which would assist you with getting a charge out of an 18 without any abundances.

Entrancing calls attention to, dietary issues or the powerlessness to control food utilization have different causes. "A few factors that could add to these dietary issues are low confidence, absence of control of life, melancholy, tension, outrage, forlornness, individual mental components.

Others are progressively relational and that can help individuals to lose control of their eating regimen at an oblivious level, for example, family issues, trouble communicating their sentiments and with spellbinding you can go to the wellspring of the issue, for this situation of food "

Eat partitions in littler plates and have measures to eat, for instance, half of the bread, half of the vegetables, of soups, either at home or in a café. Prevailing fashion consumes less calories typically cause bounce back. Along these lines it is prescribed to eat four times each day, and just when you are ravenous this can work through trance.

Through spellbinding, you can envision and devour food all the more gradually. Be evident that in the national occasions the food doesn't end ", prompted the expert.

As to with entrancing to keep up a healthful equalization, the master clarified that "it comprises of two phases. To begin with, instruct the patient, determine what it is and what is the extent of sleep-inducing treatment. Second, clarify that there is an occupation on their part.

Concerning weight control, it has to do with producing the patient a subjective alteration of their mind through spellbinding that permits them to imagine contrasts in physical and mental terms and furthermore change the dietary pattern as far as the measure of food eaten.

For this, we work with fortifications, which is the place the patient takes sound recorded by the Center for Clinical Hypnosis where there are three levels and along these lines step by step move towards another vision in regard to what it is and what we eat. "

In contrast to different techniques, the master focused on that "doesn't produce bounce back impact, it is so ground-breaking when individuals accomplish the work they choose to do what they are educated, for example, creating conduct change, mesmerizing work with fortification at home, that It is a characteristic method to see again what food is.

The bounce back impact is created in different examples. With mesmerizing, a significant change is created in the individual's conduct and impression of what they truly eat for. "

Then again, it is troublesome not to put on weight is this Christmas season, since "at any rate on normal we increase four kilos, contingent upon the special seasons".

Anyway, he gave a few hints that can help not to exaggerate the eating routine and control weight, for instance, "drink with sugar change it for one without sugar, don't utilize dressings, for example, mayonnaise or others, expend cook yet with servings of mixed greens and not with potatoes or rice, in a perfect world green plates of mixed greens that have less calories, or one day eat empanadas and one more day broiled.

The significant thing isn't to blend everything around the same time and keep away from canned organic goods on the off chance that you are going to drink liquor, attempt it with a light or zero beverage, and in this way decline the caloric admission.

Step by step instructions to Stop Overeating

Gorging is a confusion described by an urgent eating routine that keeps individuals from losing control and being not able to quit eating. Last scenes most recent 30 minutes or work irregularly for the duration of the day.

An abundance lounge area will eat ceaselessly or focusing on what you eat, regardless of whether you are as of now exhausted. Indulging can cause you to feel wiped out, blameworthy, and wild. On the off chance that you want to realize how to quit indulging, follow these means:

Keeping up MENTAL STRENGTH

Stress overseeing pressure is the most successive reason for gorging. Whether or not you know or not, the possibility is to make a complaint in light of the fact that you are stressed over different parts of your life, for example, work, individual connections, and the wellbeing of friends and family.

The most straightforward approach to lessen enthusiastic admission is to oversee life stress. This is an answer that can't be accomplished with a tip pack that can help with unpleasant circumstances.

Consider: are there certain variables that are focusing on your life? By what means can these components be limited? For example, on the off chance that you are living with an insufferable flat mate that is one of the main sources of worry in your life, it might be an ideal opportunity to escape that circumstance.

Exercises, for example, yoga, contemplation, long strolls, tuning in to jazz and old-style music can be delighted in serenely. Do anything you need to do to feel that you are in charge of your life. Attempt to hit the sack simultaneously consistently and get enough rest. In the event that you are very much refreshed, you will be better ready to adapt to upsetting circumstances.

Associate YOUR MIND AND BODY OVERTIME

You can get increasingly out of your sentiments by composing a journal that lets you compose what you have thought of, talk about your wants, and think back after a mind-boggling scene.

Taking a brief period daily to consider your activities and sentiments can hunger affect how you approach your life.

You can amaze yourself as well. You can track the food you eat except if you are fixated on each easily overlooked detail you eat. At times you can get away from allurement on the off chance that you realize that you need to compose all that you eat.

Set aside Effort TO LISTEN TO THE BODY AND CONNECT THE MIND AND BODY.

On the off chance that you recognize what your body is letting you know, it will be simpler for you to comprehend what will carry you to your outrage and deal with your eating routine. Tune in to your body for the duration of the day and give it an opportunity to have a superior thought regarding what it needs or needs.

Observe the 10-minute standard before eating a bite. On the off chance that you have a craving, don't concede yourself quickly, hold up 10 minutes, and glance back at what's going on. Ask yourself whether you are eager or longing for. In the event that you are eager, you need to eat something before your longing develops.

In the event that you have a powerful urge however are worn out, you should figure out how to manage that feeling. For instance, go for a stroll or accomplish another thing to occupy from your wants. Ask yourself whether you are eating since you are exhausted.

Is it ideal to say that you are glancing in the refrigerator since you are searching for something? All things considered, figure out how to keep yourself dynamic by drinking a glass of water. If it's not too much problem have a great time every now and then.

Keep up sound propensities Eat well suppers three times each day. This is the least demanding approach to abstain from indulging. In the event that you haven't eaten for a large portion of a day, you'll appreciate the complaint. The significant thing is to figure out how to eat the sound food you like.

So as opposed to eating what you need, you feel that you are satisfying your obligation through a dull and bland feast, your dinner ought to be nutritious and delectable.

The strategy is as per the following.

Continuously eat in the kitchen or another assigned area. Try not to eat even before a TV or PC or in any event, when you are on the telephone. There is less chance to appreciate without focusing on what you eat. Eat at any rate 20-25 minutes with every dinner.

This may appear to be quite a while; however, it keeps you from feeling when your body is full. There is a hole between the second your body is full and the second you feel full, so on the off chance that you nibble more time, you will be increasingly mindful of the amount you eat.

Every supper needs a start and an end. Try not to weave for 20 minutes while you cook supper. Additionally, don't eat snacks while making sound bites. You have to eat three sorts of food, however you ought to abstain from eating between dinners, staying away from sound alternatives, for example, organic products, nuts, and vegetables.

Eat dinners and snacks in little dishes utilizing little forks and spoons. Little plates and bowls cause you to feel as though you are eating more food, and little forks and spoons give you more opportunity to process the food.

Overseeing SOCIAL MEALS

When eating out, it is normal to expand the propensity to discharge since you feel less controlled than the earth and typical eating regimen choices. Notwithstanding, being outside ought is not a reason to appreciate gorging.

You should likewise discover approaches to maintain a strategic distance from them, regardless of whether you are in a social domain or encircled by heavenly food. Technique is as per the following.

Nibble before takeoff. By eating half of the products of the soil, you can lessen your craving when encircled by food. On the chance that you are in a territory with boundless tidbits, close your hands.

Hold a cup or a little plate of vegetables to abstain from eating different nourishments. On the chance that you are in an eatery, check the menu for more advantageous choices. Do whatever it takes not to be affected by your companions. Additionally, on the off chance that you have a major issue with bread utilization, figure out how to state "Don't include bread" or smoke peppermint candy until you have a supper.

What Is Gastric Band Hypnosis?

Gastric Band hypnotherapy is genuine and is at the present time, helping people from fluctuating foundations with their weight decline goals. These are cultivated by them and giving control in their lifestyles giving them a quick and clear way to deal with get their optimal proportion of wellbeing.

Gastric Band Hypnosis?

On the off chance that you have an in mesmerizing or hypnotherapy, by then, you have in all likelihood observed the continuous thought that trance gastric band technique has been tolerating. I will explain what they are and how they work so well.

A huge segment of you will think about gastric band medical procedure. It is the spot an inflatable silicone contraption is put around the top piece of the stomach, to help weight reduction. The circumstance of the band makes a little pocket, at the most elevated purpose of the stomach. This pocket holds around a huge bit of a cup of sustenance. (The typical stomach holds around 6 cups of sustenance.) The pocket stacks up with sustenance quickly, and the band moves back the area of sustenance from the pocket to the lower some bit of the stomach. As the upper bit of the stomach enrolls as full, it sends the mind a message that the entire stomach is full. This urges the person to be excited less oftentimes, feel full more quickly and for a progressively drawn out time period, eat tinier fragments, and consequently get fit as a fiddle after some time.

Despite the fact that this medical procedure is more secure and less prominent than other similar sorts of medical procedure, for instance, stomach stapling, it is still not without its perils. In like manner, the huge costs included are moreover a potential impediment to various people. Hypnotherapy can empty these impediments by offering another choice. Instead of continuing with this medical procedure, a clinical stupor pro can rather convince your inward brain that you have encountered this framework. They can oversee you into a trance and talk you through the procedure as if it is happening. On a cognizant level, you will realize that you have gotten hypnotherapy; notwithstanding, on a mind level, you will believe you have gotten medical procedure.

This is critical as the mind is subject for your modified inclinations. On the off chance that it acknowledges that you are not, now, prepared to eat such a great deal, by then, it will go about as necessities be. Is definitely not an issue that the aware bit of the psyche realizes that you haven't encountered medical procedure - the two can correspond okay with different feelings.

An instance of this is dreadful little creature dread. An individual can, in their wise insightful psyche, reason that a bug is nearly nothing and truly harmless. They can appreciate this amazingly well, yet their mind acknowledges regardless and establishes the customized fear response. So, an individual can, on a cognizant level, know very well that they have gotten hypnotherapy. Notwithstanding, their internal brain can totally believe it has encountered a clinical framework and go about as necessities seem to be.

A trance gastric band strategy should be conceivable at a much lower cost than medical procedure and passes on no risk. The body proceeds as in the past, and it's essentially that the mind, the part liable for modified wants and affinities, acknowledges and acts like genuine medical procedure has been done. At the point when you are eating less, the bang on effects will be weight reduction after some time. So, on the off chance that you are thinking about having the medical procedure, or you are just excited about getting slenderer, by then, Maybe the gastric trance band method is for you.

What is hypnotic belly hypnosis, and can it help you lose weight?

There is another method of losing weight known as gastric resection that has been done in recent years. It's coming to the United States from the United Kingdom and Europe, and there are some developers in progress to test how well Americans are responding to the virtual gastric banding process.

Gastric band trance uses the innovative psyche rather than the careful instrument to help overweight with peopling to recuperate control over their eating and development rehearses. You no doubt perceive what the gastric band clinical methods or weight reduction clinical techniques incorporate. The procedure is acted in a clinical facility working room where a gathering of authorities and chaperons make little passage focuses in your chest and stomach and slip little cautious instruments and cameras into your inward body. They cut and devour an entry around your stomach and join a banding contraption that would area be able to off the top bit of your stomach. The size of this top bit of your stomach can be offset with the objective that it will in general be made to get only a restricted amount of sustenance. So, you become genuinely unequipped for eating more than 4 or 5 pieces without any problem.

At the point when this cautious action is performed, on the off chance that you some way or another figured out how to eat past what your new humbler stomach can hold, you will end up being really debilitated. This is a run of the mill result that is named "dumping." It is customary to such a degree, that a word was imagined depicting the wonder. The reason behind the medical procedure is to make it mandatory for you to eat more diminutive proportions of sustenance. Tinier suppers will mean progressively essential weight reduction. There is no affirmation that you will eat smaller suppers, whether or not you have the action. Moreover, there are times when the people who have had the action have overeaten and destroyed more to themselves in light of the fact that their inward organs were changed.

This new health improvement plan, gastric band entrancing, profits by the imagery of the medical procedure. Using your inventive psyche, you will be convinced that you have had the band installed, and you will respond just as you have had the action. Your psyche is an astoundingly helpful resource for change, and your inventive brain is the route into your mistake and your triumphs. Anything that you can imagine enough, your body will respond as if it is legitimate.

So, by using the force of your brain, your stomach will feel more diminutive, and you will end up eating tinier proportions of sustenance hence. The program is also proposed to oversee and work through the reasons that you have eaten a ton already. Whether or not those reasons are affinities or sentiments, your clarifications behind gorging will evaporate. I am leaving you with the ability to amass the new affinities that will proceed your new, progressively invaluable lifestyle for an astonishing leftover portion.

There was, starting late, a few TV programs broadcasting reports about a kind of mental gastric band clinical systems. This isn't medical procedure at everything with the exception of an imaginative strategy for using your innovative psyche to empower your body to imagine that you had the medical procedure. Likewise, since your body imagines that your stomach has dried, you right now respond with feeling full speedier and declining to eat an unnecessary measure of sustenance.

This appears to be a shocking plan to various overweight people, for example, yourself, that have combat for such a long time with endeavoring to empty the plenitude weight. In the event that you perceive how our brains work, in any case, it doesn't seem, by all accounts, to be so freakish. Take, for illustration, how we respond in the current to things that we have practically identical experiences to previously.

Music is something that an impressive part of us check out reliably. Additionally, since music is something that goes all through style, we probably had checked out explicit styles of music and explicit tunes when we were significantly more energetic than we check out today. Additionally, the slants and experiences that we were encountering at that more youthful age are in all probability just antiquated accounts for us today. Be that as it may, constantly, when you check out an old tune today, it can have the effect of bringing you to the feelings, insights, and events of your life from a long time before. So, you realize how uncommonly noteworthy your imaginative brain is.

Shouldn't something be said about an experience that you have never had? By what strategy can your brain establish connections that you have no previous data on encountering? In reality, we do have certain considerations of what things would feel like, or how we would respond to explicit conditions reliant on equivalent occasions that we have encountered. We likely won't know how it feels to fly since an enormous part of us I can safely say have never influenza helped by a plane.

Moreover, in the event that you have ever watched, you likely imagined that you could fly yourself. Also, on the off chance that you use your inventive brain totally, you may have had the choice to really feel like you were flying during that dream or dream.

So, you see whether or not you have never had an experience, you can, regardless, imagine what it would feel like in the event that you did. Additionally, when you organize to use gastric band mesmerizing to help you re manage your gobbling and develop another progressively advantageous association with sustenance, you increment an unfathomable accomplice for your weight reduction.

Gastric Band Surgery Versus Gastric Band Hypnosis

So, you're thinking about genuinely stopping any fooling around about your weight issue. You feel genuinely bad, and you have to start weakening. You are certifiable to such an extent that you are as of now regardless, thinking about medical procedure to help you in dropping the weight. Since we understand that you are dead serious, we ought to go over your decisions.

Weight reduction remembers taking for littler calories than you exhaust. On the off chance that you take 3500 calories in seven days, at that point you ordinarily would, that would change over into you losing 1 pound of weight. That suggests that you should get rid of 500 calories for every day to get that moving. Through the range of a year, you will have shed 50 pounds. Augmentation the proportion of calories you get rid of from your step by step or without fail diet, and you will construct the quantity of pounds you lose as time goes on. Those are the fundamentals of weight reduction, and those nuts.

Making Lifestyle Changes for Weight Loss

It is free to say that you are attempting to get more fit. Here is the way to shedding pounds - effective weight reduction is typically accomplished by making way of life changes, not impermanent fixes. On the off chance that you change your way of life to be progressively dynamic and eat more advantageous, weight reduction falls into place without any issues. Then again, regardless of how much starting weight you may lose with a 90-day diet and exercise program, your weight will ricochet back on the off chance that you don't receive a solid way of life after those 90 days.

Submit and choose: Know that getting thinner for all time requires a pledge to better expectations of wellbeing. There is no for the time being achievement. It requires some investment and exertion and heaps of control. Focus on yourself that you are going to "gain wellbeing," not "get in shape."

Have practical objectives: Losing weight too quick isn't just ridiculous yet additionally hazardous. Set objectives that are feasible (to the extent your guidelines are) so you don't hurl the towel and give even before the finish of the primary leg of the race.

Figure out how to adore more advantageous nourishments: Reducing your calorie consumption doesn't really mean expecting to surrender all your preferred food sources. Truth be told, you can at present have your preferred dim chocolate cream cakes, as long as you stick to great solid nourishments more often than not. Keep in mind, it's a long-distance race, not a run.

Get dynamic: Pick practices you appreciate and begin organizing time to turn out to be day by day. "Exercise" doesn't mean you need to run 30 minutes on the treadmill. In any event, investing energy playing Frisbee with your children can comprise as a decent exercise. Do a little consistently, however do it. No special cases.

Get support inwardly: The exact opposite thing you need to get notification from your better half when you return from your exercise is, "Quit sitting around idly; it won't work!" If conceivable, get an accomplice for your everyday exercises to give you enthusiastic help.

That gives you more inspiration as well as makes the exercises increasingly pleasant.

Change your way of life bit by bit: We all maintain a strategic distance from change, regardless of whether it is cognizant or subliminal. Make changes step by step. For instance, on the off chance that you typically wake at 8 am and might want to get up 2 hours sooner to exercise, start by getting up 30 minutes ahead of schedule, at that point an additional 30 minutes, at that point another. Along these lines, your change will turn out to be increasingly perpetual, and you will find that the dynamic way of life turns into a propensity.

Eat Plenty of Protein

In the event that you have settled on the choice to set out on a weight reduction venture and might want to find out about the advantages of protein, at that point you've gone to the correct substance, recently I followed a high protein eating plan and lost a lot of weight. Expending nourishments high in protein is one of the most ignored pieces of a solid eating regimen. High protein nourishments offer numerous dietary advantages, critical muscle benefits for the body and can be found in an assortment of nutritious and delightful food sources. Following are only a couple of the advantages of a high protein diet:

- Protein helps keep your glucose reliable so you don't get unexpected drops in your vitality levels, as you would by eating refined sugar and handled nourishments.
- Protein helps your digestion, so you consume fat quicker! Protein takes more time for your body to separate than other food. The aftereffect of this is you will feel full for significantly more; in this manner, it will diminish your longing to keep on eating. The final product is the lower number of calories you devour; the more weight you lose!
- Protein launches your muscle versus fat's consuming instruments (the creation of glucagon), which helps with moving fat to the circulatory system to be utilized as vitality rather than been put away as fat.
- Protein is a macronutrient, which implies the body needs noteworthy measures of it to guarantee your body capacities appropriately. Protein permits the body to make hormones, compounds, and different synthetics required by the body. It

94

gives the preparation for sound blood, ligament, blood, and skin. We regularly think little of the advantage of protein, and as a rule since we essentially are misguided or don't think enough about it.

- One of the most significant segments of protein-rich nourishments is the way that proteins assemble fit body muscle. High protein nourishments that are devoured as a piece of a fair eating routine assists muscles with recovering so they can keep up their motivation and capacity with the body appropriately. Other than water, protein is the amplest substance found inside the human muscle tissue.

While picking a high protein food, know about the supplements and substances that go with that type of protein.

Nourishments that are high in soaked fats are regularly as protein, for example, red meat, so know about your decision of cut and select lean red meat.

Pick nourishments that are finished proteins and don't contain high immersed fats. Fish and poultry are normally the best decisions of high protein nourishments, trailed by dairy items and nourishments in the vegetable family, including beans and lentils.

An even eating regimen will contain an assortment of nourishments. Protein offers the human body a plenty of supplements, looks after muscle, and separates fats. Eating an eating regimen with the suitable degrees of protein will help guarantee the body capacities as it was planned.

It will likewise furnish you with the entirety of the above advantages, and whenever overwhelmed by a sound adjusted eating routine, it will add to weight reduction.

Drink Water Regularly

Up until now, you have heard a great deal of drink water to get more fit, so does the water help with weight reduction, and why? The appropriate response is straightforward truly, water helps you in losing your weight, and this is the ticket.

At the point when you make your own weight reduction plan, you first beginning by changing your dietary patterns. This is acceptable in light of the fact that the main thing you have to do is dispose of all that low-quality nourishment. Yet, many overlooks that to bar soft drink too, which makes it significantly progressively hard to get more fit.

That is the place water comes in. Rather than drinking pop, you ought to supplant it with water, and not just that, you should drink in any event eight glasses of water a day. Water resembles your normal purifier. It encourages your digestion to dispose of all that overabundance fat and calories you consume each day. So truly, water helps with weight reduction!

However, remember, water helps with weight reduction just when joined with the best possible eating routine and a great deal of preparing each day it will bring the needed outcomes. Particularly after you've gotten done with some broad working out, you have to drink a lot of water. Water will assist your body with getting free of the considerable number of poisons and fat that you have recently consumed.

The procedure is troublesome, and numerous before all else can't clutch this arrangement. The motivation behind why this is being to such an extent that toward the start, your body is attempting to dispose of all the overabundance water in your body, it has been putting away water every one of those years since it was worried about the possibility that that the water admission may stop because of the unpredictable water supplies.

Furthermore, since you have begun with the standard admission, your body won't hesitate to dispose of all the negative and exorbitant water in your lower legs, for instance. Along these lines, your body is currently confident that there is no compelling reason to flexibly any water and flush the extra away. There is a valid justification why water is extraordinary and helps a great deal in your eating routine. To begin with, it enables your body to dispose of all the negative segments that your admission, and afterward it is calorie and sans fat. Whatever other juice that you may drink holds calories that you in the end need to consume. With water, which is in some cases called harmful calorie food, you don't have that issue.

Your body needs to warm so as to process the water. Since water is o calorie nourishments, you are consuming more calories. What's more, that is the reason water assists with weight reduction.

Eating more vegetables

Taking loads of vegetables will diminish your weight the manner in which you have never thought; dissimilar to protein vegetables are light, which may not get you topped off rapidly, stop your feeling hungry for a considerable length of time. It's a verifiable truth vegetable just little starch. Also, simultaneously give an incredible wellspring of fiber and nutrients. The entirety of this will assist you with losing weight quick without work out.

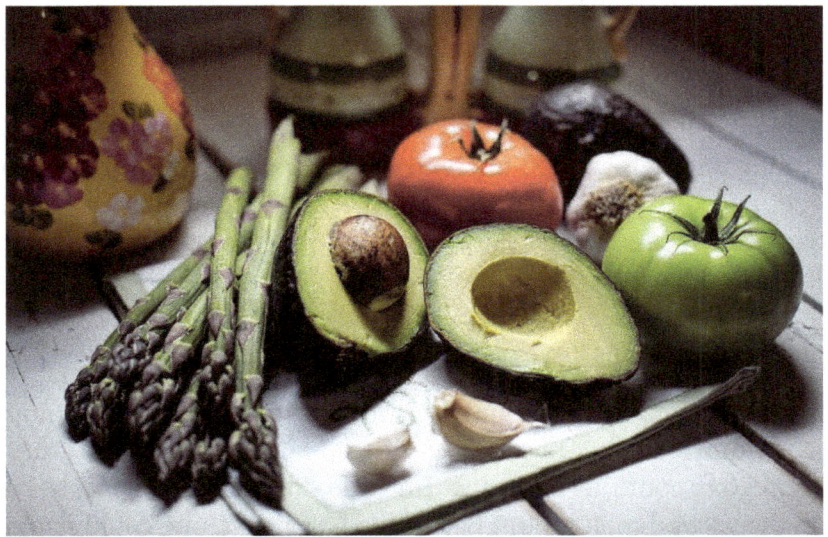

Past Life Regression Hypnosis

There is a catchphrase in spiritual circles, and if you don't know it, you may be ashamed as I was the first time, I heard it. The saying goes: You are not a body that has a soul; you are a soul that has a body. The message here is that the body is transitory, and the soul is eternal.

Think about the consequences of this for a second. If the soul is eternal, then all and all materials will survive. The universe can go back and forth; however, we will be here. This is only the main surprising thing, the way that once the spirit starts to exist, it can never stop to exist. It follows then that we will live great lives and almost certainly, in the billions of long periods of the universe's history, we have just lived innumerable lives.

Some consider it to be a type of heck, the spirit is constantly dedicated to returning and living again in some material manner, totally without recollections and along these lines inclined to living a similar catastrophe again and again. They look to the eventual fate of the planet and think: "The future won't be useful for people, so how might it be useful for the spirit? How might it be useful for individuals who will resurrect as individuals later on? "

There is additionally an increasingly critical view. The world is brimming with agony and wretchedness, so a spirit that is compelled to return is always forced to continue suffering. Imagine this: a soul that existed like an ox in the second millennium BC. In the Near East, one could imagine that it was a difficult life for an ox. Now imagine that the same soul returned as a woman to Athens in the 5th century, or as a slave to a Roman estate in the 2nd century BC. C. What about these other cultures that have collapsed from disease, famine, and war? It would be difficult to say that the existence of souls during these periods was a significant step from their previous lives. All of these lives seem to be treated with misery and reduced quality of life.

Now imagine if this happens more often than not. After all, for most of human history, many people have suffered, lived short lives, been malnourished, were illiterate, inferior, and have always lived in some

98

form of confusion, as the forces were always in conflict with each other. or facing instability. Nine out of ten people lived in the lower class, as farmers or less, for much of history (Ponting, 2000). This is certainly different from now on when nations fight less, and most of us eat well, have heat, and have access to unimaginable luxuries like clean water, medicine, and other technologies that have transformed our lives. Compared to life for most of human history, the average person today, since industrialization, lives like a king. It then follows that the souls that began to exist as human beings from the beginning of civilization until now had more bad lives than good ones.

What this argument for eternal torment forgets is that things have gradually improved, and not only that, human history itself is but a blow compared to eternity itself. Eternity is how long it will be. If things always improve, in eternity, the greatest tragedy that humanity can experience will not compare with other levels of existence that await our souls in the future. They are unthinkable by the standards we have today. So, in essence, even if things were terribly terrible for us here on Earth, for each of us, that would be nothing compared to eternity.

And if we've already lived thousands of lives, it makes sense that some of them were wonderful, some weren't that great, and some were just fine. Life is very complicated, and it goes from good to bad, and it is beautiful. People who suffer are not always unhappy and miserable.

Every life we start is like a new role given to an actor. We take on this role with purpose, purpose, and mission. But before the actor realizes it, he forgets who he is and begins to think that he really is, and always has been, the character he plays. Forget that the role it plays is only for this movie, for this result and only for that purpose.

This is what happens in our souls. We forget that this is a role for many that will determine our entire career, give it meaning and shape. An actor is not judged just for the big part and judged by his filmography. The only paper is like a canvas brush. There is still a lot to do if you want to compete with a memory. You can imagine how sad it would be if an actor forgot who he really is, but for many of us, this happens.

We live without knowing who we were, what our current life is like, and therefore we are prone to suffer or even be hampered by past life experiences that manifest themselves in various ways, such as depression, irrational phobias, compassionate reactions, appall in certain things without valid justification, stress, constant torment and substantially more.

The body we have now, with its natural interruptions and a brain that is exceptionally worried about its place in another job than with its job in the comprehensive view, is only a show. The objective of previous existence entrancing is to free you up to significant previous existence encounters that have happened during your excursion into this universe, encounters that include importance, setting, and course to your encounters now. He will do it, so you don't lose focus. You will be progressively rebuffed, recognizing what to stress over and what not to stress over. You will know without a doubt what your most noteworthy concern ought to be and what does not merit your vitality or consideration. It will give your life extraordinary harmony, which means, and a feeling of direction.

The primary working material of past life entrancing is creative mind and contemplation. All mesmerizing utilizes the psychological procedure of the brain. Consider subjective procedures as apparatuses of the brain. The brain takes care of issues and works through different psychological procedures, for example, thinking, memory, judgment, recognition, structure, and then some (Cherry, 2019). The primary prerequisite and totally essential part for the entrancing activity of the past life is the creative mind. You don't need to be very phenomenal or innovative.

Odds are you've lived incalculable lives, and the same number of you will see as you experience sleep inducing meetings, you will have a wide assortment of encounters, some of which will stand out from others. This is to be expected. You have lived many lives, you have many memories, and you have played many roles. But all this will be important to your place in the world right now, and that is why your higher self, your deeper self, or your spiritual guide show you these memories. It allows you to access them because they are related in some way. You will not always know why this is so, but you will see it again. It will become possible for you as you go through your life, and the more you do, the more things will materialize, and most will be explained or illuminated by your hypnotic journeys. If you hear something like this for the first time, you may be wondering what a spirit guide is. Some call them angels. These are entities that do not need to be angels, who are in charge of guiding their role on Earth. Basically, they're here to make sure things run smoothly, that you're living a life that allows you to move on to the next. They are intangible, spiritual, and often communicate with us in various ways, usually when we are in altered states of sub consciousness, such as dreams and trans. Of course, this is not the only time this communication has taken place. It consistently appears in countless ways. We just have to be much more open and perceptive. They would not be excellent caregivers if they only spoke to you in altered states of consciousness. What shows to be occurring is that people are learning to ignore or suppress the various signals that come their way as they move through their busy lives. As a result, they feel lonely when they are not. Intuition is one of the most popular ways of doing this, but there are other ways.

There is a story I heard about a subject who was experiencing acute physical pain on her left shoulder. The pain was unbearable, and nothing seemed to make it better no matter what she tried. She had chronic pain, and no one knew what was causing it. She was told that it was all in her head. Nothing she was given would help with her pain. She discovered, in a past life regression hypnosis session, the source of her pain.
It turned out in her past life, she was a man who had died in battle, and someone had hacked her left shoulder. For some reason, she had not let go of that trauma going into this life. She was the same age when she died then as she was when the pain started. Knowing this allowed her to make peace with had happened to her, it allowed her to deal with it head on, and with that the pain gradually subsided until it was entirely gone. It is possible that many of the things we struggle with are remnants of past life trauma we are having trouble letting go of. This is just one example of what past life regression hypnotherapy can do.
Some of you might be listening to this with skeptical ears, not knowing if you should take any of this seriously or believe it. Perhaps you believe

in some other conglomeration of beliefs that dispute anything like past lives. And that is okay, too. The benefits of past life regression session are not only for those who do believe in the phenomenon. They are open to anyone who is willing to try. Transcendental and vivid experiences aren't closed to you either. Anyone can experience them and derive meaning and value for them. For you to experience this, for you to take away something handy from this, you don't have to believe in my ontology.

Ontology refers to the philosophical study of what exists. Ontological statements are those that assert the existence or non-existence of something (Inwagen, 1993). Within my ontology are things like souls which are eternal and live countless lives. But perhaps your ontology and worldview are starkly different, denying any existence of immaterial things like souls. Your ontology might only conceive of human beings as a bunch of atoms arranged in precise ways to produce life and consciousness as we know it.

Maintaining Your New Weight Loss through Hypnosis

Have you ever had the reality of being so successful at losing weight after being a member of a weight loss club for a few months, only to regain all the weight you lost when you stopped looking regularly?

It almost seems like a conspiracy that will make you pay to keep going to the weight loss club. Otherwise, you may not be able to maintain your weight loss.

So, to be successful, you must do more than simply go to a weight loss club or follow a diet routine in a newspaper.

It's about changing your mindset about your weight and perfecting that diets work. Yes, if you follow what is written or what they have told you and you will lose some weight. However, weight is in many cases and most cases come back very quickly once you decide to go back to a "normal" diet. If diets don't give you a good result, what can you do to be the way you want to be and stay healthy?

Eat regularly: You may have tried to shed weight by skipping meals entirely. This does not work because your blood sugar level drops and you begin to crave a lot of sugar and other simple carbohydrates. As a result, you will eventually find yourself eating too many calories, high fat, and unhealthy foods, and as a result, you will find that congratulations come back too quickly anyway.

Eat healthy: If you think it's really what you're eating, and you're trying to make your diet as healthy as possible without being a fan, then you're much more likely to be able to control your weight by controlling your mind.

A healthy diet means a balanced diet, eating plenty of fresh fruits and vegetables, low-fat protein, healthy fats like olive oil and avocado, and also many complex carbohydrates. It also means cutting down on foods that contain sugar and white foods like white flour, white rice, and white pasta and instead of eating more food throughout the meal.

Relax often: If you tend to eat more when you feel anxious, take a few minutes when you feel anxious to close your eyes and breathe slowly as you inhale and exhale at any intensity.

Listen to your body: Learn to listen to what your body tells you it needs at any time of the day and allow yourself to have what it looks like, even if you know the healthy guidelines mentioned above.

Drink green tea routinely.

Bunches of individuals have just borne witness to for the medical advantages offered by green tea. It helps your stomach related framework in preparing the nourishments that you eat. All the more critically, it is additionally found to have gainful impacts in forestalling malignant growth, because of its poison battling segments.

Eat more organic products.

Organic products are stacked with natural nutrients and dampness to keep you feeling better. It is perhaps the ideal approach to forestall ailments and blockage. Most organic products additionally contain chemicals that help your body in engrossing the supplements offered by the nourishments that you eat.

Tips for Great and Healthy Living

The ideal approach to accomplish better wellbeing is to change your way of life. It's tied in with causing a change from the nourishments you to eat to the exercises you do in your regular day to day existence. You can begin by staying away from lousy nourishments, slick, and handled food sources, since they will include more pounds into your body just as start setting aside some effort to work out. This will empower you to have a better capacity to burn calories, which will help consume more fats just as get your body fit as a fiddle. This is only something you can do in remaining sound. To get more direction, simply read on as right now, we share with you tips on how you can begin your way towards a more useful life and you! Appreciate!

1. Sleep for at any rate of 8 hours every night.

Having enough rest part of the most significant activities to improve and keep up your wellbeing. It can make you increasingly vigorous the following day, besides the way that it can likewise forestall binge eating. All the more significantly, it is additionally perhaps the ideal approaches to prevent diseases, since it toughens your insusceptible framework.

2. Wash your hands as often as possible.

Washing your hands for the same number of times as you can for the entire day is perhaps the most ideal approach to forestall diseases. It ought to be finished with running water and a decent antibacterial cleanser. What's more, washing ought to be accomplished for in any event 20 seconds, to guarantee that it is liberated from any malady disease germs.

3. Never skip breakfast.

If your objectives are to get more benefits and to abstain from putting on an excessive amount of weight, at that point, skipping breakfast ought to be the keep going thing on your mind. Breakfast is the essential meal of the day. The feed can prop you up all consistently. If you skip it, odds are, you would put on weight because of binge eating and limited capacity to burn calories.

4. Drink, at any rate, eight glasses of water every day.

Water can help your body in flushing out poisons. Besides that, it can likewise guarantee that you are appropriately hydrated. Besides, drinking water can also help in stifling your hunger, which results in a fitter you. In this manner, make sure that you drink at any rate eight glasses of water each day to keep up your wellbeing.

5. Limit espresso consumption.

Espresso can now and again influence the nature of your absorption, which is the reason it ought not to be drilled all the time. A great many people drink various cups of espresso every day. To get more benefits, it is ideal if you chop it down to only one container for each day, or just to make drinking espresso a trivial thing.

6. Purchase a littler plate to either chop down your weight or to look after it.

Decreasing the measure of nourishments that you eat in every meal can have an emotional impact, with regards to keeping up or shedding pounds. Something you can accomplish for it is to buy a little plate, which is for your utilization as it were. With a bit of dish, you can fool yourself into eating littler segments, which would give you bunches of medical advantages over the long haul.

7. Try not to eat whatever isn't on your plate.

To acquire control on the measure of nourishments that you eat every day, it is ideal to abstain from eating nourishment that isn't on your plate. There are loads of occasions when you might need to get a bunch of peanuts out of the holder or take a sample of soup out of the bowl with a spoon. If you keep on doing this, at that point, you include more calories into your body without knowing it.

8. Eat-in a slower way.

Eating quick is probably the ideal way if you need to put on more weight. Like this, you are doing something contrary to that can result in losing an abundance of pounds of weight. In this way, the time has come to make the most of your meals more by eating more slowly. At the point when you eat more slowly, you can stifle your craving, and it can likewise cause you to feel full, regardless of whether you have not expended a lot of nourishments yet after a specific timeframe.

9. Be sound emotionally.

As opposed to what a few people may accept, your feelings likewise assume an incredible job with regards to your wellbeing. In this manner, it is ideal if you can oversee it. As such, attempt to forestall blowing up, and consistently attempt to have an uplifting viewpoint of life. At the point when you do this, you can get more settled in most testing circumstances.

10. Think positive.

A few people may not trust it, yet your mind can influence your wellbeing in specific manners. For instance, if you generally imagine that you are becoming ill, at that point, it would build your odds of getting influenced by an ailment. Then again, if you believe that you are stable, at that point, you become increasingly dynamic, and it would likewise support your insusceptible framework.

11. Dodge popular fashion diets.

Most craze diets are diet programs, which are intended to cause individuals to get more fit quickly. By and large, these projects can include causing the individual to experience starvation, which can result in a quicker rate in getting more fit. In any case, because of the way that it has been accomplished, you can restore the weight in merely an issue of weeks, and you may even get heavier than when you previously began with it.

12. A brisk stroll for 3 to multiple times every week.

Energetic strolling is a movement that you can appreciate with your loved ones. It can help in boosting your digestion, which can result in weight loss. Besides that, it can likewise take care of business, your hips, bottom, just as your legs. Intend to energetic stroll for at any rate 20 minutes in 3 to 4 times each week, to pick up the advantages from it.

13. Exploit practice recordings.

If you are the sort of a person, who wouldn't like to invest energy in driving, to find a right pace rec center, at that point, remind yourself that there are practice recordings that you can exploit. These recordings can be played at the solaces of your home whenever you need them. You should simply follow the schedules appeared in it and appreciate them.

14. Play with your children all the more frequently

Children are so lively, and we regularly wonder why. Be that as it may, if you play with them, you can help your vitality level too. This can result in a higher metabolic rate. In this manner, it can assist you with consuming more fats and calories, besides the way that doing it all the more frequently can likewise give you an approach to bond with them more.

15. Drink a glass of water when you wake up.

Drinking a glass of water after awakening offers a ton of medical advantages. For one, it gets your framework working, which can support up your vitality level. What's more, it can likewise help in purging your assemblage of poisons that have been aggregated for a long while.

16. Sharing is something that you ought not to do in ensuring your wellbeing.

With regards to your wellbeing, sharing ought not to be finished. This relates to the sharing of your things to different people, for example, hankies, toothbrushes, nail cutters, and such. The facts demonstrate that sharing is acceptable. However, this ought not to be watched about your own things.

17. Mind your pets.

A few people don't know that there are sure ailments, which can be transmitted from creatures to people. Along these lines, if you have pets, at that point, ensure that they are given their suggested inoculations. What's more, you ought to likewise make sure that they are appropriately prepped, with the goal that they are liberated from ticks and bugs that may also convey germs.

18. Try not to confound ache to hunger.

There are periods when we open up our coolers to get a bite, in any event, when our body is aching for water. This is because we tend to decipher thirst as appetite. Consequently, if you want to eat in any event, when you have quite recently had your meal, at that point, attempt to drink a glass of water. By and large, you will feel fulfilled as a result of it, particularly since you were dehydrated in any case.

19. Maintain a strategic distance from prepared nourishments as much as you can.

Handled nourishments like franks, burgers, French fries, and such don't contain enough supplements to furnish your body with what it needs. Besides that, they are likewise topped off with a ton of artificial flavorings, which can make your body amass bunches of poisons. Therefore, it is ideal for evading them for as much as you can. Staying away from them can help forestall maladies, besides the way that it would likewise help in making you more beneficial.

20. Eat nourishments that are high in fiber content.

If one of your wellbeing objectives is to shed a couple of pounds, at that point load up on fiber, fiber draws out the absorption procedure, which implies that it can cause you to feel full more. At the point when that occurs, you usually are stifling your hunger. Besides that, fiber can likewise help in freeing your assortment of waste.

21. Cut down your utilization of carbonated sodas.

Carbonated sodas are stacked with a great deal of sugar, which can make you put on weight, and it can even build your odds of getting diabetic. A few people who are partial to drinking such refreshments incline toward diet ones since they guarantee to contain lesser measures of sugar. Be that as it may, such beverages are stacked with aspartame, which can cause heaps of medical problems over the long haul.

22. Utilize the stairs rather than the lift.

At whatever point you report to your office, make it a propensity to utilize the stairs rather than the lift. This can offer an original route for you to consume more fats and calories. It is a type of activity, which can fortify your leg muscles, and it is a decent option in contrast to running or lively strolling.

Additional Tips to Help You Lose Weight

Now, if there's one thing many people are still dealing with in the world today, it's unnecessary weight gain, which is triggered by too much fast food. But with the aid of your side's fitness book, and a few ideas you can try out you will significantly reduce your body's excess fat to give you the youthful look you've had in the past.

While it is a process that takes some time, if you need to get rid of your new body stance at all, you, as the victim, will demonstrate a lot of persistence as well as discipline. And what are some of the tricks with the fitness manual by your side that will make you lose weight within the shortest amount of time? The first thing you can work out is to eat a lot of fruits and vegetables and minimize fat-rich foods.

Having that in mind, you should have a routine follow-up practice that you can do, including taking a short stroll, if you find it challenging to perform rigorous workouts. This will encourage you to eat very balanced foods and do a few light fitness manual exercises from the guidebook.

The other advice is to eat healthy, organic meals, which will contain more vegetables and fruits, and drink green tea after every heart-warming meal you take. This method is very successful, specifically for those who prefer slimming down the natural way. Less calorie intake would also significantly help to decrease the bodyweight because too many calories in the body begin to slow down the body's metabolic process, thereby contributing to the weight already gained.

This is one difficult decision that many people may not be gracious enough to take, but it is the only way out of the weighty issue. Besides, if you choose to consume fewer calorie foods and perform different fitness manual exercises, then your vital body metabolism rate will bounce back into shape faster than you expected. Did you notice that drinking a lot of water will help you lose weight quickly as well?

When you're on a strict diet to lose weight, the body needs to be hydrated all the time to maintain its optimal levels and reduce the excess weight gain and water retention that might be present in the body. You're good to go, with a little fitness boost. Many tips to help you lose weight faster include eating potassium-rich foods, calcium, routine workouts using the fitness guidebook or video, a healthy diet plan, and a positive attitude throughout.

Forget the anguishing stories you read about how tough it is to lose weight. Make it easier for yourself to help you lose weight by following these ten quick and easy tips. Implement one tip every day, and you'll be at your target weight before you know it: no hassle, and there is no need to turn your whole world upside down either. Don't waste any more time on medications and expensive treatments or hard-earned cash, start to use these tips today and also be lean and healthy.

1. The first trick to help you lose weight is to have healthy eating habits. In this way, you can not only obtain more food quantity, but you can also use natural low-calorie seasonings such as onions to enhance the taste. It is known for long-term wellbeing and weight loss as the diet burden itself is eliminated.

2. Trim the fat always off the meats that you cook. Or if it is chicken-like, cut the fat. Chop it up and add it to something like pasta, if that is too bland!

3. Get a friend accountable for your diet program. People tend to be more committed after a week or two when they know and need to check in with others. For starters, find someone to walk with, a close friend or even a diet-boyfriend. Say your goals! Sometimes trying to do something by yourself can be a lot harder.

4. To keep track of calories, carbohydrates, proteins, etc., write down everything you consume. You would be shocked if you didn't write down your menu, how many extra items you would drink. Either plan with your dietary intake or start keeping a food log to see!

5. Using a non-stick canola cooking spray, if you need to fry stuff. It will save you plenty of calories over oil cooking. One tablespoon of cooking oil, for example, contains 120 calories! Considering that a 2.4-second PAM spray contains just 16 calories.

6. Keep the outlook optimistic, and never give up. When/if you leave, is the only time you struggle. It may take further work or some other strategy, but it will "will" happen. Studies indicate that the majority of people struggle to try their first time. Nothing

will take the place of determination! Not intellect, not talent, absolutely none! All the rest is secondary.

7. Their diet and wellness programs are 50/50 partners in the weight loss program. When one or the other is missing, you'll have less chance of success! You can workout until you pass out, but you would not see drastic improvements in your appearance if you take too many calories in. And if you don't do exercise, the body is more likely to use muscle rather than fat for energy. Aerobic exercise causes fat burns! Hunger burns up fat!

8. Reflect on the loss of fat and not just the overall weight loss. What matters is your size, and not how much you weigh. You may be surprised because the muscle is more substantial than fat! So know calories burns with the muscle! So, eat meals regularly and don't miss it. When you wait for more than four hours, your metabolism will start slowing down.

9. Know where fat appears to get the body. Women seem to accumulate fat around their thighs and glutes. Men gain it on their bellies and around their waist. This is because of the lack of circulation in those regions. Fat isn't taken as quickly into the bloodstream as other regions. That's why fat burning agents such as ephedrine work alongside a long-term weight loss plan. Help even to blood-thinning agents such as aspirin. Still, before using any replacement, make sure you read the labels, directions, and alerts!

10. Keep your weight loss program clear. If you start missing meals or skipping workouts, it slows your progress to the point of discouragement. How bad do you want that to happen? Select and stick to a good plan. Know, what you put in you gets out of it!

Most people are becoming more conscious of their weight, not just because of how it impacts the way they look but also because of the consequences of their wellbeing. If you're one of those looking to get a leaner body, you certainly should be entertaining the simple but successful techniques.

Turn Your Back on the world of fast food.

Of course, ordering food from a drive-through or over the phone is more relaxed, but if your heart is set to lose significant weight, then this is the

112

first step towards achieving such a goal. You'll have to start eating at home as an option, or if you're a busy person and can't handle such a job, you can always eat at restaurants that have a healthy menu on offer. Turning your back on fast food will also mean giving up processed foods like crispy chips and carbonated drinks.

Apply more liquids to your diet.

Water is a significant factor in the weight loss cycle since it is the carrier of all the nutrients from the food you consume. Keeping this in mind, make sure you drink at least 8 full glasses of water a day, as well as a few glasses of fresh fruit juice. Citrus fruits and berries make excellent shakes because they taste fantastic, and they contain a lot of antioxidants too.

Find the Right Weight Loss Supplement Though – Some people are vehemently opposed to using all kinds of weight loss aids, such as fat-reduction tablets, but having a little boost is nothing wrong. Nonetheless, it is imperative to choose the correct form of supplement and to steer clear of "quick fix items" that are currently very common on the market.

Dedicate 1 hour per day for exercise.

Allot at least one full hour for cardio, no matter how busy you are at home or work. If you have home gym equipment, you can produce quicker results as you can work out daily. An alternative would be to run around your neighborhood block every day for a total of 30 minutes to an hour.

10 Weight Loss Myths

I will open the top weight reduction fantasies in the briefest answers with the best potential beneath:

Have you at any instance felt like you were doing everything that you were being advised to do to lose the additional pounds? Indeed, you are not the only one. The media controls such a large amount of your reasoning now and again it is hard just to settle on the correct choice. There is a big deal of data on the planet on weight reduction, yet all of us battles with settling on the correct decisions. The legends are the most elevated misguided judgments I have found in my vocation of 15 years as an expert mentor. Use them quickly to your everyday schedule. To have achievement you must have the correct data, yet you will likewise require the assurance and inspiration. You hold the force in you to begin now.

Fantasy 1-If, I work out with loads I will get enormous and massive

The best way to get enormous and massive is to keep on having awful dietary patterns. You have to discover your resting digestion. What amount of food do you have to devour to be sound, shed pounds, and feel extraordinary? You need to make a decent attempt on any individual to get your muscles to develop. It is the exact opposite thing to stress over. Concentrate on utilizing a lot of muscles a day to work out to consume the most extreme measure of calories. A recouped muscle will consistently beat a worn-out muscle. That implies less calories consumed for you if your muscle is drained.

Fantasy 2-Just doing cardio will give me the best fat consuming outcome.

Despite the fact that cardio represents heart lungs. It doesn't mean the most remarkable fat killer. Truth be told, the harder you push your body at a time or exercise with a similar exercise the almost certain of utilizing your muscle tissue for vitality versus fat stores. See fat consuming in the 3-day window. Not today. Regardless of whether that program worked. The most significant drawback would be that your lungs extend to another level EVERY 10 minutes. That implies from the entire first day you begin losing your capacity to consume as much fat...If, you can't make sense of why you have thin legs. It could be from an excessive amount of running. That may crash your digestion. To what extent can you really be a long-distance runner? Some may attempt, and yet, it isn't likely you. It requires some investment to prepare for a long-distance race. We are talking 50 miles every week! Also, the mileage on your connective tissue. I am not against long runs. It feels better. It's simply not my entire course of action.

Fantasy 3-You have to work your entire body each day

Your body needs an ideal opportunity to change. Your body does the entirety of its supplanting and dropping while you are snoozing. Around 90% of any outcome happens when you are rest. Not when you are wakeful.

Your body will adjust to any exercise you do each day. Quick adjustment will warrantless outcome. You need to pick an enormous and little muscle bunch every day. Assault it with a great deal of vitality. Wash and rehash that procedure week by week. At the point when you return week by week you will be more grounded. Giving you a superior fat consuming exercise each time. A lot of overtraining happens when you do similar muscles or activities consistently.

Fantasy 4-Liposuction will offer me the response I need

Actually, you will more than likely be directly back to where you began. What? How is that? All things considered; your plastic specialist can indeed remove a limited amount of much at once. More often than not that enchantment number is a WHOPPING ten pounds. After your medical procedure, you can't move for 3 weeks. I couldn't care less what they let you know. I have seen it again and again. Since you can't do anything your body eases back down. In this way, anything you eat remains with you. I have seen individuals really put on weight. Have not met one individual that said they needed it once more. Also, that you have rub or back rub your wounds, so water doesn't get caught between your skin.

Legend 5-Fat is awful for me

The truth of the matter is fat has two implications. One is the caring you eat. That has a couple of various names inside that. At that point their body fat. Cells or fat tissue. They are not the equivalent. Your muscle to fat ratio is put away food. With perhaps some water. End of inquiry. The body couldn't care less whether is it's a sugar, protein, fat, or whatever else the body didn't consume off.

115

Dietary fat has taken negative criticism. In my eyes and 15 years of experience-fat is genuinely not even our concern with our nourishments. Truth be told, you will require fat in your body on the off chance that you would prefer not to age rapidly, or you need to drop muscle to fat ratio, keep hormone levels offset, fix muscles. Something else, your body is feeling the loss of individual bits of the riddle. It isn't adjusted. It manages no doubt convey a more significant number of calories per gram than the other significant macronutrients. They are the carbs and proteins.

Fantasy 6-All starches are awful for me

You will require them to adjust your blood sugars. Which is the way to dropping muscle versus fat and vitality? Not notice not feeling discouraged. In the event that, you do a no-carb or ketogenic diet you will discover genuine snappy what it resembles to feel like soil without carbs. You don't need to do this!

Continuously know how your food is reaped. At that point what occurs on each stop of its way to your table. On the off chance that it was initially earthy colored and now it is white, something is absent. To the body, it isn't a similar food any longer. The name of the food doesn't make a difference. Your body separates food. It very well may be called wheat bread, even have shaded added to the bread, and on the off chance that it is prepared and faded. It isn't the equivalent. Good wheat won't cause weight gain. It won't cause weight gain.

Prepared weight will quite often cause weight gain.

It is free to say that you are beginning to see the image.

Fantasy 7-Rice, wheat, and grains are terrible

It doesn't make a difference the sort of food it is. It is crucial what befalls the glucose once you eat the food. The regular buyer purchases food that is separated as of now or is utilizing sugar for an additive. The two hot weight control plans out Paleo and crude vegetarian neither eat any sort of handled food. Let the light glimmer for a moment. Alright. Earthy colored rice is your companion. For whatever length of time that it isn't moment.

Fantasy 8-Red meat is awful for me

It is the thing that the meat has been handled in is what is awful for you. Perhaps it has been siphoned brimming with hormones. At the point when you add white prepared bread to an overwhelming handled fat. That is your mix for a respiratory failure.

Without a doubt the most noteworthy food in nutrient and is red meat liver.

A burger from the cheap food spot can get you in a difficult situation. It has been vigorously prepared in all manners. Saved and over-prepared.

Fantasy 9-Your digestion is moderate

That is another word that has various implications. Your digestion is your capacity to separate your food. Putting away your food is another procedure. The slower the food separates the to a lesser extent a possibility there is to store that food, or some would call it vitality.

In all likelihood your body separates food fine. Indeed, I have never observed a particular situation where your body doesn't separate the food accurately. There are different circumstances that may cause issues. At the point when somebody meddles with your hormones that can dramatically affect weight. Exactly at all cost avoid playing with hormones. Your body will get diverse by then. All the more critically, you may consistently be stuck taking that hormone or thyroid prescription.

Fantasy 10-I just need to concentrate on my calorie admission.

Indeed, the measure of food you expend affects your capacity to lose fat. The sorts of food are similarly as significant if not increasingly significant. What your body does with the food once it is inside you is the genuine inquiry. Will your body consume this food or does your body need to fix? On the off chance that, not it will store. I have seen firsthand when an individual gets a lap band and get incredible outcomes. Eating less 1000 calories every day. At that point following two or three months, the body adjusts to that 1000 calories. Presently, what are you going to do?

A lap band is a band around your stomach that is carefully put there. It stops your signs to need to eat. It makes your stomach littler. Ensure you put the sort of nourishments before the amount of food. Encircle yourself with the best possible sorts of food.

What is Reflection?

Reflection is a type of preparing that interfaces the mind and body to achieve a sentiment of calm. People have been considering for an enormous number of years as a powerful practice. Today, various people use contemplation to diminish weight and end up being dynamically aware of their appearance.

There are various types of reflection. Some rely upon the usage of clear articulations called mantras. Others revolve around breathing or keeping the cerebrum at the present time.

These methodologies can help you in working up an unrivaled cognizance of yourself, including how your mind and body capacities.

This extended care makes reflection an accommodating instrument for better understanding your dietary examples, which could realize weight decrease. Scrutinize on to get acquainted with the benefits of reflection for weight decrease and how to start.

What are the upsides of reflection for weight decrease?

Contemplation won't cause you to get slenderer medium-term. In any case, with a little practice, it can possibly and adequately influence your weight, yet moreover, your idea design.

Prudent weight decrease

Contemplation is associated with a variety of focal points. With respect to decrease, care contemplation is, apparently, the steadiest and practical. A 2017 review of existing examinations found that care contemplation was a convincing procedure for getting progressively fit and changing dietary examples.

Care contemplation incorporates giving close thought to:

• where you are

• what you're doing

• how you're feeling at this moment

During care contemplation, you'll perceive these points of view without judgment. Endeavor to view your exercises and insights as essentially those — nothing else. Consider what you're feeling and doing yet take the necessary steps not to gather anything as being lucky or tragic. This gets easier with normal practice.

Practicing care contemplation can incite great stretch advantages, also. What's more, interestingly with various wellbeing food nuts, those contemplation care will undoubtedly keep the weight off, as demonstrated by the 2017 review.

Less Shame and Disgrace

Care contemplation can be particularly helpful in controlling enthusiastic and stress-related eating. By getting progressively aware of your insights and sentiments, you can see those events when you eat in light of the fact that you're pushed, rather than hungry.

It's in like manner a not too lousy gadget to shield you from falling into the risky twisting of disrespect and accuse that a couple of individuals capitulate to when endeavoring to change their dietary examples. Care reflection incorporates seeing reality with regards to your slants and practices, without settling on a choice about yourself.

This urges you to pardon yourself for submitting blunders, for instance, stress-eating a pack of potato chips. That exonerating can moreover shield you from catastrophizing, which is a luxurious term for what happens when you decide to mastermind a pizza since you are starting at now "failed" by eating a pack of chips.

How would I start reflection for weight decrease?

Anyone with a mind and body can practice reflection. There's no prerequisite for any remarkable apparatus or exorbitant classes. For a few, the hardest part is mostly finding the time. Endeavor in any case something reasonable, for instance, 10 minutes out of each day or even every other day.

Guarantee you approach a serene spot during these 10 minutes. What's more, since you have adolescents, you may need to squeeze it in before they wake up or after they head to rest to restrict interference. You can even have a go at doing it in the shower.

At the point when you're in a quiet spot, make yourself pleasing. You can sit or rests in any position that feels basic.

Start by focusing on your breath, seeing your chest or stomach as it rises and falls. Feel the air as it moves all through your mouth or nose. Check out the sounds the air makes. Do this for a second or two, until you start to feel progressively free.

Next, with your eyes open or shut, follow these methods:

1.Take a full breath in. Hold it for a couple of moments.

2.Slowly inhale out and repeat.

3.Breathe regularly.

4.Observe your breath as it enters your noses, raises your chest, or moves your waist, yet don't transform it in any way.

5.Continue focusing on your breath for 5 to 10 minutes.

6.You'll find your psyche wandering, which is absolutely standard. Essentially perceive that your mind has wandered and return your respect for your breath.

7.As you start to wrap up, consider how adequately your mind wandered. By then, perceive that it was so typical to return your thought to your breath.

Endeavor to do this a more significant number of days of the week than not. Recollect that it most likely won't feel incredibly amazing the underlying barely any events you do it. Be that as it may, with ordinary practice, it'll get more straightforward and start to feel continuously standard.

Distinctive consideration systems

Here are two or three distinct tips to help you with receiving a consideration-based system to weight decrease:

•Slow down your meals. Focus on gnawing step by step and seeing the kind of each eat.

•Find the helpful chance to eat. Keep away from eating in a rush or while playing out numerous errands.

•Learn to see craving and totality. What's more, since you aren't energetic, don't eat. In the event that you're full, don't forge ahead. Endeavor to check out what your body is telling you.

•Recognize how certain sustenance cause you to feel. Endeavor to concentrate on how you feel in the wake of eating certain sustenance. Which one's reason you to feel tired? Which one's reason you to feel engaged?

•Forgive yourself. You felt that half quart of solidified yogurt would make you feel good, yet it didn't. That is OK. Increase from it and continue ahead.

•Make progressively shrewd sustenance choices. Contribute more vitality pondering what you will eat before truly eating.

•Notice your wants. Requiring chocolate again? Perceiving your wants can help you with restricting them.

Use a mantra that causes you get increasingly fit.

A mantra is a word or articulation that you admit to yourself to focus your preparation and return you to center when your psyche wanders. As Libshtein explains, "a mantra can give you something to focus on while you think." Although various people feel that its steady to their preparation — especially since you pick something that impacts you before long — it is by no means, essential. Do whatever it takes not to feel like you need to constrain yourself to use one since it doesn't feel typical or pleasing. What's more, since you choose to use one, Libshtein prescribes repeating it to yourself as you take in and again as you inhale out. Standard choices join "I am revered," "I am settled," and "Om." If a mantra mostly doesn't feel legitimately for you, Libshtein says to focus on your unwinding simply.

Follow your breath to reduce pressure.

"Give using four counts a shot as you take in and eight counts before you inhale out," Libshtein suggests. Nevertheless, contemplation is connected to reducing pressure, so if these checks feel pushed or unnatural, it's OK to stray from them. Endeavor to manufacture your counts each time you reflect. "Make an effort not to be concerned and in light of the fact that it requires some speculation to work up to eight checks," Libshtein says. "Basically, understand that extending the inhale will basically help calm you down."

Endeavor a guided contemplation for weight decrease.

Feeling to some degree lost without any other individual? Try not to stress over it! There are a ton of records, computerized accounts, locales, and phone applications that partner you with pros who can guide you through reflection rehearses until you feel great going just it. Libshtein's site, Mentors Channel, is just one instance of such a help.

What might it be prudent for you to foresee from doing guided reflection for weight decrease?

What's more, since you have to use reflection expressly to get fit as a fiddle, look for guided contemplations that consideration on that as their subject. The ace in the video or sound record will most likely demand that you imagine a couple of things: what you may intently look like after you've lost the weight, a rousing person who has quite recently made sense of how to get progressively fit and what they may think and feel, what they apparently never really get fit as a fiddle and keep it off, and how you can solidify these penchants into your own extraordinary consistently life.

Are there hindrances to using contemplation methods for weight decrease?

Contemplation should be seen as just one instrument in the entire weight decrease tool stash. Diet and exercise are critical bits of the condition too, and you're persistently going to see the best results when you join all of them three into a lifestyle that you can continue with long stretch. The key with reflection, like check calories and exercise, is duty. You need to remain with the preparation to see suffering changes. That is the explanation we offer 21-day programs, so you can see changes that as a general rule last.

You ought not fight it, you ought to fundamentally bend it to their will, overpower it, teach it.

Exactly when your accomplice is nothing, or nothing, it will be impossible for you ...

Likewise, contradicting before a donut or another cheeseburger or not wanting to locate a useful pace to the rec focus will be a breeze.

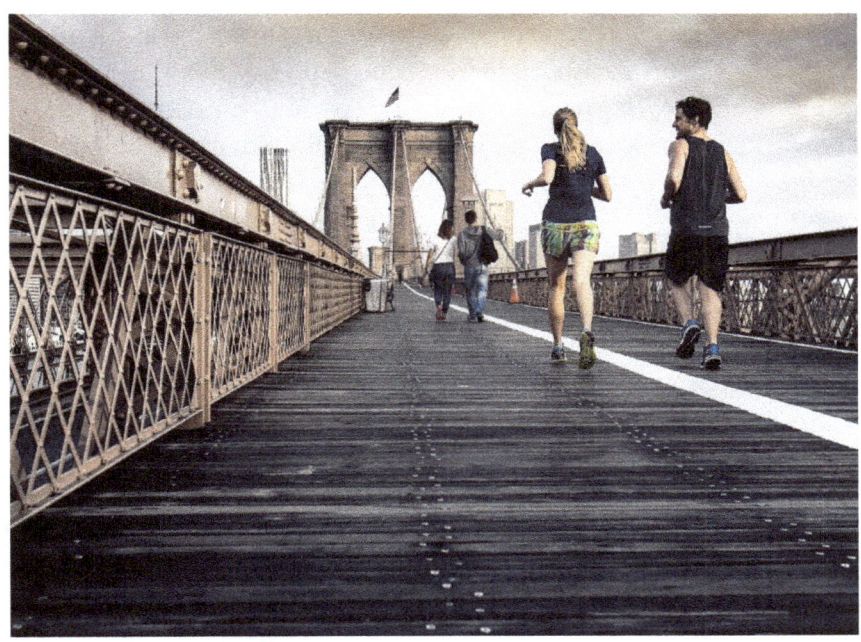

Healthy Body

Plan to enter a covert government of unwinding. Start by altering your body into an agreeable position. Set down. Loosen up your legs and spot your arms out at your sides from your body with your palms up. Tenderly close your eyes. Take in a moderate delicate full breath. Breathe out gradually. Take in once more. This time hold your breath for a second until you hear me state discharge it. At the point when you let the breath out this time, envision that any negative contemplations emotions or energies are coming out of your body. Do that presently... discharge it... great. Take in a considerably more profound breath and hold it again until I state discharge it.

Envision you're taking in quieting loosening up vitality. Letting out pressure and strain and discharge it. Great. One final time all alone. That is acceptable. Your breathing is loosening up you. For the rest of this meeting, each breath you take starting now and into the foreseeable future will keep on loosening up you more profound and more profound. Take one more breath with me. Cause your body to feel looser than before you took that breath. Take in and loosen up further and let it out. You are much more profoundly loose than previously.

You have molded your psyche to have the option to unwind on order principally by taking in and setting your goal on unwinding. You're making a robust situation inside and all around your lungs as you keep concentrating on taking in this essential sound manner you're doing well at this point.

How about we take this unwinding you're encountering somewhat more profound, center the entirety of your consideration around your pulse. Tune in and notice the mood of your pulse. Put an image of your heart in your inner consciousness. See it beating in an ordinary sound manner. Notice how stable your pulse is. At the point when you loosen up along these lines and inhale profoundly all the time you reestablish all the cells in your body to their natural solid state. The progression of the oxygen currently present in your body, makes you discharge pressure. You're turning out to be quiet and progressively serene. You assume responsibility for your life at this moment and the entirety of the progressions you need to make by basically unwinding and connecting with that piece of your psyche that makes whatever you want. You're setting aside a few minutes for this every single day. You appreciate this time. You appreciate dealing with yourself on each level; intellectually, inwardly, genuinely, and profoundly.

Keep on concentrating on your breathing now and consistently. How about we take this unwinding a little more profound presently by concentrating the entirety of your consideration on your eyes. Concentrate eagerly now on your eyelids and you're going to make your eyelids become loose with the goal that when I instruct you to and not up to that point you will attempt to open your eyes and discover you can't.

In the first place, we will get them loose. Free and limp. Free and limp. So, loosened up that you won't have the option to open your eyes. Your eyelids are getting stayed together. Your eyelids are starting to feel like one bit of skin. Your eyes won't open regardless of whether you attempted. Need that to occur. Get that going.

In a second, you'll get the opportunity to discover exactly how fantastic your brain truly is. You will attempt to open your eyes and find that you can't. While remembering you realize you could open your eyes in the event that you needed to. At this moment, they're feeling too worn out too loosened up that they need to remain shut. Presently attempt to open your eyes and find that you can't. Invest somewhat more energy. Quit attempting and unwind. Loosen up your eyes. Go further. More profound loose.

To go considerably more profound loose, I will recommend that you open and close your eyes a few additional occasions. Each time you open your eyes and afterward close them once more, you will twofold your unwinding.

Presently, open your eyes. Close your eyes and go further, much more profound. Once more, open your eyes and close them once more. Twofold your unwinding. Twofold your unwinding... Go significantly more profound. Once more, open your eyes and close them. Dive deep. Let your body totally let proceed to unwind.

Each muscle in your body is totally free and limp and this feels better. Your brain is ground-breaking when you accomplish this degree of unwinding. You permit yourself to stay at this profound degree of unwinding basically by concentrating on the sound of my voice and the ambient melodies. While you might have the option to recognize some different sounds, any sounds that may commonly upset you will just relaxingly affect you.

Whenever you notice any sounds around you, they just motivation you to go further loose. Simultaneously, my voice will impact your psyche mind in an impressive manner. My voice will go into the most profound degrees of your inner mind psyche to make the progressions you want to make in your life. My voice will consistently animate a loosening up alleviating quieting feeling inside you. So, you will promptly start to connect my voice with unwinding the second you start to tune in. You will see yourself having the option to accomplish further degrees of unwinding each time you practice.

(Discretionary symbolism)

Permit your psyche to take you to a delightful spot. A spot you pick that is sheltered and warm and agreeable. A spot out in nature... A spot that makes and much more profound feeling of quiet and harmony inside you... Take a second to make this different spot.

Since you've made this unique spot, envision you are resting on the ground. Notice your degree of association with this spot. You currently extend your degree of association basically by taking several moderate full breaths. Notice the way that the ground underneath you empower your body. What a mind-blowing feeling to feel the very life power vitality of the universe streaming within you. Reestablishing your body to consummate wellbeing.

As you take in picture you are taking in the environment around you. Each breath you take causes the hues you see around you to turn out to be increasingly transparent, splendid, and pleasant. As you watch out into the inaccessible sky, you will see a rainbow. You permit each shade of the rainbow to mix together and structure one segment of white light that compasses down from the sky and contacts the highest point of your head. Feel the way this light feels.

As it fills the highest point of your head, unwinding, mending light. Purifying each cell in your body as it keeps on streaming down from the highest point of your head and into your temple. Streamlining the little space between your eyebrows. Spreading out through your whole face, your nose, your cheeks, your jaw, and your jaws. Loosening up each muscle and nerve. Feel this light descending your neck. The rear of your neck... The front of your neck... Retaining any pressure and snugness.

Feel this light descending into your shoulders, loosening up your shoulders. Let your shoulders become free and limp. Feel this loosening up vitality going through every one of your arms, your hands, and down to the tips of your fingers. From your neck and shoulders down into the top piece of your back. Going down and around every vertebra and into your lower back. From your neck and shoulders down into your chest and your midsection and your stomach. Loosen up your stomach muscles. Loosen up your stomach muscle totally.

Feel this influx of vitality reaching out into your butt cheek muscles. Discharging and loosening up that zone totally... Your thighs feel this vitality. The muscles inside your thighs are unwinding. Your knees, your calves and into your heels... Feel this vitality gathered into that one focal area, your heels. Move such vitality into the curves of your feet. Feel it in the bundles of your feet. Your toes... You have used this mending light to loosen up you totally. Presently send it out from your toes down into the ground as you recollect where you spread out in nature.

Negative Emotions and Weight Loss

We all have emotions though some people are more emotional than others. They are called feelers. Emotions refer to the way we handle or react to our feelings.

Behavior is mostly influenced by brain biochemistry rather than logic. That is why when we let our mind wander and take control of our brain, then we can enjoy the weight loss benefits of meditation. Human beings are emotional, thus can be rational. This is why, when stressed, addicted, or overwhelmed; it will not matter on the best advice they get. Chances are at that particular emotional state; they may not act on the information. The emotional brain thus is right to say that it always has more precedent than the rational brain. The ability to rationalize almost every behavior makes us able to persuade ourselves. This makes us believe that we can do anything that we put our minds into. This makes it hard to convince ourselves to do the things we don't want to do and will come with all sorts of excuses to justify that. Weight loss is significant to your health and general physical well-being. The psychological impact of rapid weight loss may have an adverse effect on your mental health. The need for abrupt weight loss surgery may not give your mind time to prepare for the changes, thus causes severe psychological problems. Meditation, however, gives your body and mind time to adjust the intended body change, thus making you emotionally ready when that time comes.

The human body is an essential and excellent tool that is made to regulate self and heal. It is what we have for a lifetime. So, it is our duty and responsibility to look after it well and ensure that it does not malfunction. So many books have been written about weight loss through diet. However, food has not been useful for everyone and sometimes can even cause stress if the diet is not working. Meditation, however, is a stress-free proven method that is effective and sustainable. It also guides you into eating what you want when you need it without the unnecessary guilt or restriction to a particular diet. Meditation can protect you from the world of emotions and offers an effective way of handling overweight excuses. Through this, you can learn to take responsibility for your life choices and be ready to face the consequences. Do not suffer in silence, if something is not going on as expected; open up and confide to someone safe from your group or a professional psychologist. Stress or emotional discomfort can sometimes affect our appetite and our response to challenging situations whenever you internalize negative emotions ranging from anger, disgust, fear, prejudice, and others. It is your body that processes all these things, and sometimes your body clings to them long after the incident is gone and done with.

Depression

When one is exposed to excessive stress, and they are not able to deal with it, they will be at risk of getting depression. It is a mental illness that affects millions of people across America, and some victims have to depend on anti-depressants to survive. Meditation comes in handy since diet-induced weight loss has been linked to depression. People who have weight issues and are attempting to lose weight in vain have low self-esteem and are likely to look upon themselves and not appreciate their worth. Depression can be associated with reduced motivation, and self-efficacy will hinder one's ability to achieve their set goals. Depression affects so many people, and if mismanaged can lead to madness, suicide attempts, and bodily harm. Depression causes a lot of strain on the nervous system; thus, the quietness and harmlessness of meditation can be a start of the healing process. When one is depressed, they will blame themselves for their predicament, they will not know what to do and will be surrounded by a lot of self-guilt. Meditation provides the necessary assurance that you are not the one to blame, and nothing is your fault. Meditation helps you create your purposes, escape previous failures, and start again for your good.

Stress and Anxiety

When one is stressed and anxious, they may overeat or under eat depending on the circumstance, either way, this will lead to severe weight issues. When one tries to lose weight in vain, also they may be subjected to emotional stress. This is if they do not have the needed support system at their disposal. These negative emotions make one not to be productive and sometimes make them hopeless and not see the value of life. Hopelessness can prevent one from doing productive things that make life meaningful. It makes one even hate the simple hobbies that once made them so happy. Mediation, however, creates that you need to connect with the activities that you enjoy doing, whether with your friends or alone. When you do things, you love, you will be happy and find a new meaning in life. You will indulge in the things that are productive and add value to your life.

Eating Disorders

This comes about when there is high pressure to lose weight in order to look more appear in a particular way. Women are more likely to be affected by eating disorders compared to men. This is because women to go on a diet in order to lose weight. Eating disorder, if not treated, can pose a severe health risk and bodily harm. Too much eating can cause obesity. Overeating when negative emotions set in can cause bulimia while not being able to eat for fear of being fat can cause anorexia. Meditation frees your mind and lets you be free to eat whatever you want but being limited to healthier food. Negativity, if not dealt with, can cause permanent emotional health issues of the body. Meditation helps prevent eating disorders or help cure an eating disorder for people already affected. Eating habits are controlled by the mind, which may not be easy to explain sometimes. The mind triggers some emotions, which in turn helps one get off binge eating.

Dealing with Negative Emotions

- Face up to old pains and hurts. Sometimes, previous hurtful experiences leave a permanent wound in our brain. Are there some of the things that you were told that you still bury in your chest? How did those words make you feel? It is essential to let go and move on. These hurts can cause permanent trauma and thus cause permanent emotional damage, which is not healthy for one's health.

130

- Be free to express yourself. Keeping emotions to oneself can lead to inner turmoil build-up, which in turn leads to an unexpected or involuntary reaction to the daily situation. If you are not an expressive type and find it hard to express your inner emotions, then consider keeping a journal. This will help you release some of the stress-energy wills that might interfere with the general well-being.

- Reach out to people. It is important not to always depend on people for validation or approval. However, when negative emotions come up, it will, therefore, be essential to reach to people, it can be a trusted friend professional in that particular field. There are proven therapies like; talk therapy and hypnotherapy, which are very useful in dealing with stress issues as well as removing negative emotions.

- Be kind and at peace with yourself. Emotions are powerful, but your mind is often in control. Sometimes depending on the situation, it may not be easy to control your emotions. When things go out of hand, remember to be kind to yourself. With this regard, we can control how we react to different emotional scenarios. Reward yourself as you respond well to negative emotions and appreciate your effort to create and maintain an atmosphere of peace.

- Feel your best to look your best. Unwanted weight gain can be hard to address; however, if you fail to discuss what's going on in your mind, you may not feel worthy. Your body is naturally designed to protect you. Thus, you should feel free to release inner feelings troubling you and be ready to get help. Being in control of your emotions will help you feel good and appreciate yourself as a whole.

- Putting too much emphasis on our emotions can sometimes hinder our success. While some people know how to control themselves during stressful situations, others have developed a coping mechanism where they cannot allow negative emotions to bring them down. It is okay, however, to freely express our emotions and let the teardrops fall when we feel sad. Suppressed emotions cause trauma, which in turn leads to poor eating habits, thus might cause rapid weight gain or weight loss. Emotionally unstable people also are often irritated, not focused, and may get into fights a lot.

Impact of Negative Emotions on Diet

- Negative emotions can cause a lack of appetite. This is a state where one does not have the urge to eat despite feeling hungry. Loss of appetite may be due to too much distraction, and when the mind is not settled. Sometimes one will feel like eating, but when food is presented before them, the urge to eat disappears. Loss of appetite can also be experienced during sickness, which can also bring negative emotions. Simple meditation exercises can calm emotions and speed up the recovery process.
- Anorexia. Negative emotions can contribute to this kind of disease. People who have been bullied because of their weight and so stop eating at all will get anorexia. They will be very thin, pale, and often tired. Severe cases are experienced when one chock themselves so that they can vomit the food they had eaten. To them, they associate food with the bad experiences they had undergone.

Guided Imagery

Trance, entrancing isn't done continuously by an individual to another. There are ways that an individual could spellbind himself. Here, the individual presents himself, loosens up himself and gests spellbound without anyone else. This technique, where the subject is being recommended or taught without anyone else, the subliminal piece of him will have no issue or damage in tolerating the recommendation made at all, which makes the strategy the best one, as it is significant in entrancing that the subject and the trance inducer or the educator place abundant confidence on themselves. Considering the way that here, in this self-trance, the subliminal specialist and the subject are very much the same, there will be no issue of confidence! So, this technique is frequently picked by numerous individuals who are looking for inward unwinding and are happy to persuade themselves for a superior future.

Self-entrancing is only the endeavors put by oneself to unwind or quiet themselves. Self-trance is utilized widely in present day hypnotherapy. It can appear as spellbinding completed by methods for an educated daily practice. Spellbinding may help torment the executives, tension, and despondency, rest issue, corpulence, asthma, and skin conditions. At the point when this training is aced, it can improve fixation, review, upgrade critical thinking, reduce cerebral pains and even improve one's control of feelings. During self-entrancing, an individual is typically taught to rehash or murmur a word, over and again over and over to himself until his psyche becomes quiet.

Individuals who are attempting to escape a specific way of life, individuals who are attempting to embrace another, improved propensity are the most widely recognized clients of this treatment. Heavy drinkers, individuals with dietary problem, individuals who are happy to leave the medications past them will discover this amazingly valuable and making a difference.

How to?

Presently that you've realized what is and what are for the most part the advantages of self-trance, you should get familiar with the strategy utilized for self-entrancing.

To begin the procedure, you have to feel genuinely loose and agreeable. Sit, rests level on stomach, or lie on your back, anyway it satisfies you. Take a stab at utilizing a basic unwinding procedure, for example, the one laid out on our Relaxation Techniques page. Discover an article that you can concentrate your vision and consideration on – in a perfect world this item will include you looking somewhat upwards on the divider or roof before you. Away from brain everything being equal and simply center around your article. This is clearly very difficult to accomplish yet take as much time as necessary to let contemplations leave you. Become mindful of your eyes, consider your eyelids getting overwhelming and gradually shutting. Concentrate on your breathing as your eyes close, inhale profoundly and equitably. Reveal to yourself that you will loosen up progressively every time you inhale out. Slow your breathing and let yourself loosen up further and more profound with each breath. Utilize your inner being to envision a delicate all over or sideways development of an article. Maybe the hand of a metronome or a pendulum – anything that has a standard, gradual swing. Watch the thing influence in reverse and advances or here and there in your inner consciousness. Delicately, gradually and drearily include down from ten in your mind, saying I am unwinding after each number. '10 I am unwinding'... '9 I am unwinding' and so on. You can even recurrent the expressions of your solace, similar to, your own strict conviction. Accept and advise yourself that when you complete the process of checking down you will have arrived at your sleep-inducing state. At the point when you have arrived at your entrancing state the time has come to concentrate on the individual articulations that you arranged. Concentrate on every announcement – envision it in your inner being, rehash it in your considerations. Remain loose and centered. Unwind and clear your psyche again before bringing yourself out of your entrancing state. Gradually however progressively vivaciously tally up to 10. Invert the procedure you utilized before when you tallied down into your trancelike state. Utilize some positive message between each number, as you check. '1, when I alert I will feel like I have had an entire night's rest' ... and so forth. At the point when you arrive at 10 you will feel completely alert and resuscitated! Gradually let your cognizant psyche find the occasions of the day and keep feeling revived.

What is Guided Symbolism?

One other method in self-unwinding is Imagery. Guided symbolism is a self-improvement or restorative mediation during which an individual pictures thing recommended so as to make physiological and mental mending. Guided symbolism, as a strategy utilized in self-entrancing encourages you in the Reduce pressure and improve wellbeing, Increase profundity and speed of recuperating, upgrade health, stir mindfulness, develop sense of pride, fearlessness, and confidence, advance innovativeness, Inspire top execution for you and your family.

Imagine a lemon. Picture you are grasping the lemon. Picture it obviously in your psyche. You can see its shading, feel its rough surface, and see the stem. Imagine that you drop it on a wooden table and hear the sound it makes. Picture you have a sharp blade and are cutting the lemon in two. See the cut surfaces shimmering and notice that you have even sliced one of the seeds down the middle. Presently imagine a shining clean glass and crush the juice from one of those parts into the glass. See it run down the side of the glass.

Presently picture that you are lifting the glass towards your face so you can smell the lemony kind of the juice. Spot the edge of the glass in your mouth and as you tilt the glass up, let the lemon juice stream down the side of the glass into your mouth. Taste the lemony taste. Taste the acridity of the juice as it streams over and around the sides of your tongue. Appreciate the tart flavor and notice the progression of salivation.

This is the means by which Imagery works. The contemplations and pictures you hold in your psyche throughout the day have impacts at subliminal degrees of the mind and can cause changes in your body, your conduct, your sentiments, and you're thinking. Also, careful this method, we will in general change the musings and supplant them unusual ones. Not exclusively does the guided symbolism, representation, and self-trance help to make another mood and in this manner experience of "reality" which sends a correspondingly unique quieting substance message to the body, yet in addition the procedure includes strengthening positive considerations or thoughts and positive conduct changes or activities. The new helpful self-proclamations and perceptions truly support, inspire, propel, and invigorate; instead of dishearten, feed cynicism and uneasiness, and decrease vitality and activity, as the negative ones had done.

Using this device and procedure to decrease pressure and enter a casual state upgrades your resistant framework, lessens the negative effect of stressors on your body (counting improving specific medical issues), reinforces your capacity to react in a useful and productive manner to life's difficulties, passionate burdens, physical and enthusiastic requests - all because your body and psyche's assets are done being depleted by incessant and additionally exceptional pressure or strain. It is an enabling procedure: information in addition to compelling instruments and the aptitudes to utilize them gives your capacity to make change, take care of issues, and achieve what you make progress toward.

- Negative emotions can lead to rapid weight gain and in turn, causes bulimia. This is when someone starts to find comfort in food. They have a constant need to eat and cannot stop themselves from eating. As they eat, so does their weight increase. They may gain weight that they will not be able to lose if given a chance immediately.

Developing comfort in a certain kind of food. Sometimes when one is exposed to negative emotions, they tend to find comfort in particular food that makes them feel good about themselves. This food can lead to overindulging the bring bringing about rapid weight gain. Comfort foods are a number in making someone add unnecessary weight.

Hypnosis for Irritable Bowel Syndrome

Take yourself to a place where the time required to complete the process won't bother you. Ideally, sit up straight, with your feet flat on the floor and your arms outstretched, without touching them. Then follow this step-by-step guide.

Cause hypnosis using a method of your choice.

A progressive relaxation procedure for hypnotic entry works well with this session, as IBS patients benefit from additional physical relaxation.

Tune into your insides. First, simply move your sensitization to your general intestinal tract.

How you feel; Is there traffic? Is there sound? Coordinate for a few minutes and focus attention and awareness on your intestinal tract. As you focus on this, let your breath relax and watch your gut respond to your soft breathing.

Just focus on the abdominal area as you breathe, allowing each breath to keep you focused and aware of your abdominal area. Once you begin to relax and feel that you are in tune with the gut, continue with the next step.

Step three:

Start imagining your gut as a flowing body of water. It could be the flow of a spring, stream or waterfall (choose the one that suits you best). Begin to imagine that the flow of water is warm and relaxing. Go back to this step to create the perfect water flow and imagine your gut as this flowing body of water.

Tell yourself that your running water sinks deeper into hypnosis and deeper into your mind, and then continue with the fourth step.

Step four:

Change the speed of the water flow to meet your personal needs. If you have constipation, make the water flow as fast and vigorously as necessary.

If you have diarrhea, let the water flow decrease. Check the flow of soothing water. Once you have determined the correct and most useful velocity for the flow of water, take time to observe and enjoy the flow at that velocity.

Then, once you've tuned in and enjoyed controlling the rhythm of the water, continue with the next step.

Step five:

Repeat your breathing and the entire intestinal tract. Concentrate on that and now let the regulated flow of water begin to heal and calm down.

Allow the water to begin to relax and warm the entire stomach, large intestine, intestines, and intestines, spreading warmth and soothing sensations throughout the abdomen. You can imagine that water has color. You can imagine that water has sound. Observe how it feels in the abdominal area as you imagine the warm, relaxing and smooth sensation of healing water flowing at the correct rate but relax with your breath and spread it to all of you.

Spend as much time as you want in this step. Enjoy it, enjoy the control you have and when you have spent enough time enjoying the warm and relaxing sensation of the water, then go to the next step.

Step six:

Now accompany these beautiful feelings with positive and reinforcing knowledge. Repeat a progressive personal enhancement to enhance the warming effect. Use your internal dialogue and repeat something to yourself: "I feel relaxed" or "my stomach becomes more and more relaxed" or "each breath I breathe calms and relaxes my stomach area".

Also, keep in mind that comfort, relief and feeling of control is something that stays with you after this session. Also, repeat to yourself that each time you use this technique, it works cumulatively better and more reliable for you and that you reap more benefits as you practice it.

Really incorporate your knowledge, use your internal dialogue consistently and convincingly, and then continue to the next step.

Step seven:

You can spend more time relaxing the area with lukewarm water, and then when you're ready, come out of hypnosis by counting from one to five.

There you have it, the first in a series of IBS self-hypnosis and treatment tools: remember that repetition is king of these procedures, and the more you practice it, the better the results.

Using a warm hand to facilitate IBS

Following the above procedure, follow another simple and easy procedure to treat IBS symptoms.

We all know for sure that when we have undergone a tummy tuck, we often instinctively place our hand on it as a means of relief, just as a parent might have done when we were younger. Similarly, when I was in my teens, I remember being in bed with stomach cramps after exercise and dehydration. I found a hot water bottle in my stomach to help him relax, stop spasms, and finally soothe him. pain.

This hypnosis session is similar to the previous one in that it helps to relax and alleviate the stomach area from the symptoms of irritable bowel syndrome. It also helps create a sense of self-efficacy in treating these symptoms and gives us a sense of personal control. Ideally, when we begin testing these types of procedures, they can be used not only as a precautionary measure. Still, they can also be used as skills to treat and treat symptoms if they occur in the future.

Get comfortable, careful, sitting or lying down (if sitting, ideally with your feet on the floor) with your arms and legs spread out. Make sure your dominant hand is palm up, then we are ready to go.

Just follow these simple steps:

Step one:

Cause hypnosis using the preferred method.

Second step:

Focus all your attention and all your consciousness on your dominant hand that has the palm facing up. Imagine that the area in the center of the palm begins to heat up. Just start with a small heat spot in the middle of the palm, and then imagine it spreading and expanding, slowly, firmly, and surely.

There are several ways to use your imagination to help you with this.

First, you can imagine a hot water bottle being placed in this hand as the heat spreads throughout the hand.

Second, you can imagine that heat is a color that you associate with heat and that color spreads.

Third, you can control when you were on an open fire with the lights on, remember how the glow felt. Imagine that your palm is held in place by such extraordinary lateral interests and you think the infamous heat gently spreads over the palm of your hand.

You can choose to use another method to imagine that your hand is warm and pleasant. Reveal to yourself that your hand feels warm, combined with your imaginative soul all the time.

Let me believe and, while it happens, let me take you to the depths of your mind. Just when you have a commendable certainty and a conclusion of warmth in your hands, which predicts that you need to relate to your imaginary mind and recognize and hold on to it, until then go to the accompaniment stage. Stage three:

Ideally, you should simply force yourself on your elbow, move your warm hand, and place it on your stomach. At the convergence point of your stomach.

With less effort, move your warm hand to the stomach area. At the point where it will appear, begin to imagine how hot it is when it comes in contact with the stomach area. Start spreading the heat and relax the feeling of recovery in the stomach area. Imagine invading your stomach,

140

stomach related organs, assimilation pathways and various zones, warming up, relaxing, relaxing.

Once again, it's essential to let your innovative soul go wild, whether it's the secretion that runs through your insides, or the apartment that brought boiling water to your stomach, or the glow it brought from the coals to calm down, to relax. and warm up significantly. - Engage your innovative soul in the way that suits you best.

Put a lot of vitality into this movement and keep doing it until you notice a glow in your stomach that relaxes and reduces the stomach area.

Stage four:

Continue to relax until you rest, warm up, and calm down. As you do this, start using your internal discussion and insight to improve and improve this method. Be sure to use heat, touch-up, and relaxation resources. For example, "My stomach is progressively free" or "I am getting a load of these heat sensations while piercing is easier."

Be sure to declare it with the end goal you are agreeing to is refreshing and reliable and to such an extent that it checks out the warm and relaxing atmospheres that get to your stomach and incorporate local settings.

At the point where you said it and repeat it over and over to strengthen your resources, take the appropriate step.

Stage five:

Sometimes, you will make a mental figure out of being in a situation in your life, probably a situation that you have generally avoided in the face of stress at IBS points that are expanding and causing problems.

Imagine being in this situation and feeling these reliable warming resources in your grip, calming down, warming up and releasing your stomach in one area, keeping your stomach progressively lovely and free, in a stable state. Imagine being in this situation and feeling warm. Start combining the brightness and the feeling of relaxation you have for this meeting with the land you imagine.

This requires a short time and peace of mind to be careful so that you can benefit more from this concentration. Reveal to yourself that you understand that you are showing signs of progress in this strategy and that wherever they need you, you can use your warm hand to calm and release the stomach area. The old and unfortunate symptoms will diminish and diminish.

Not if, ands or but fascinating. Confirm your confidence in your ability to do this when you need to, and then go to the accompaniment stage.

Stage six:

Immediately begin to imagine that the glow of relaxation begins in the stomach area. It begins to spread throughout the body. Engage in unique relaxation as you let this warm sensation spread from the warm areas of your stomach all over your body. To accomplish this, choose any procedure you have done in the past, using relaxation that activates rest.

At the point where you have expelled your entire body, proceed substantially to the last development.

Stage seven:

Leave the ecstasy by dialing one to five.

Keep your stomach warm, if necessary, and continue to increase your confidence.

Calories and Weight Loss

What's a calorie?

A calorie is a unit of vitality. Verifiably, researchers have characterized "calorie" as a unit of vitality or warmth that could emerge out of an assortment of sources, for example, coal or gas. In the wholesome sense, a wide range of food — regardless of whether fat, protein, starch, or sugar — are significant wellsprings of calories that individuals need to live and work.

"Our cerebrum, our muscles — each cell in our body — expect vitality to work in its ideal state," said Jennifer McDaniel If we don't get enough of the supplements [that calories provide], there are adverse outcomes, regardless of whether it's losing slender bulk, not having the option to think, or not getting the vitality we need every day."

In an increasingly linear structure, calories are characterized as:

A calorie is a unit of vitality. In sustenance, calories allude to the vitality individuals get from the food and drink they devour and to the vitality they use in physical activity.

Calories are recorded in the wholesome data for all food bundling. Many health improvement plans focus on lessening calorie consumption.

What number of calories should individuals devour day by day?

What number of calories an individual devour in a day relies upon the degree of movement of the individual and the metabolic resting rate that can be determined at a specialist's office or a dietitian's office, McDaniel said? "There is tried and true way of thinking that men ought not to devour less than 1,500 calories and that ladies ought to eat 1,200 calories to guarantee an equalization of significant supplements and micronutrients."

The National Institutes of Health (NIH) gives rules on calorie prerequisites to different ages and levels of movement. A moderately aged, decently dynamic female can eat 2,000 calories each day. A

143

moderately aged, modestly dynamic male can eat 2,400 to 2,600 calories for every day.

What should those calories be?

The Official Dietary Reference Intake (DRI) distributed by the National Academies of Science, Engineering, and Medicine prescribes that 45 to 65 percent of calories should originate from sugars, 20 to 25 percent should originate from fat and 10 to 35 percent should originate from protein. Youngsters need a higher part of fat, somewhere in the range of 25% and 40% of their calories. Close to 25 % of the total calories are required to originate from included sugars.

McDaniel said that past these general rules, the measure of macronutrients required relies upon the person's activity level. For instance, a competitor needs more sugars. Food inclinations additionally have a task to carry out.

What are fatty nourishments?

Nourishments that are viewed as high calories, or calories thick, have high calories to their serving size, as indicated by look into Oils, spread, and different fats; seared nourishments; and desserts are fatty nourishments. While unhealthy nourishments are frequently connected with shoddy nourishments, some are additionally high in supplements.

Solid nourishments high in calories incorporate avocados (227 calories for each cup), quinoa (222 calories for each cup), nuts (828 calories for each cup of peanuts), olive oil (119 calories for each tablespoon), entire grains and, with some restraint, dull chocolate (648 calories for every bar) as indicated by the USDA Nutrition Database.

Raisins are a case of a fatty tidbit that could confound a few people; you may expend 1 cup of grapes and get an equal measure of calories from a one-quarter cup of raisins, as indicated by the Mayo Clinic. Dry natural products are generally thick in calories; in this manner, they are well known among explorers consuming consume a lot of calories.

What is low-calorie food?

144

Nourishments considered low-calorie have a low-calorie comparative with their serving size. Foods grown from the ground, specific, vegetables are normally moderately small in calories. For example, 2 cups of destroyed romaine lettuce or spinach have 16 calories. An enormous stem of celery has ten calories, one huge ear of corn has 123 calories, 1 cup of broccoli has 15 calories, and orange has 70 calories, as per the USDA Nutrition Database.

What are unfilled calories?

Void calories contain next to zero supplements. As per the USDA's Choose My Plate battle, they regularly originate from included sugars and strong fats. Strong fats set at room temperatures, for example, margarine, shortening, and grease found in certain meats. They can normally happen yet are generally added to nourishments.

Numerous nourishments have a lot of void calories. Nourishments, for example, sausages and hotdogs as instances of mainstream nourishments high in void calories. A portion of these nourishments, for example, cheddar and pizza, likewise contain supplements (cheddar is high in calcium and contains protein; pizza sauces, fixings, and hulls can have supplements) while different food sources,

For example, soft drinks and most confections contain just void calories. Pick My Plate to name such purge calorie nourishments.

Calories and weight reduction

Although it's essential to expend adequate calories, checking and cutting calories can enable numerous individuals to shed pounds. Calories are consumed through physical movement. For instance, running a mile could consume around 112 calories following Runner's World Magazine. Research shows the calorie devoured and calories consumed as a caloric rate. It works like a scale; when you're in harmony, the calories you expend are adjusted by the calories you consume. This implies you will keep up your body weight. As indicated by the CDC, on the off chance that you are dealing with your weight, you are in caloric parity. This implies each day; you are generally devouring a similar measure of calories you are consuming. In the event that you are in a caloric overabundance, you are eating a larger number of calories than cooking, and you will put on weight. On the off chance that you are in a caloric shortfall, you are consuming off a larger number of calories than what you are eating, and you will get more fit.

Most occasions, when individuals need to get in shape, they endeavor to have a caloric shortage. Indeed, even an individual with a shortage of caloric requirements to devour enough calories to capacity and remain solid. Eating enough calories oversees bulk during the weight reduction process. It likewise enables make to weight reduction reasonably. "On the off chance that somebody slices calories to lessen weight, what occurs from that point? Does it mean they continue eating less and less?

Expending adequate calories during the weight reduction is likewise indispensable to keeping up a solid metabolic rate.

Cutting and tallying calories for weight reduction

Tallying and cutting calories can likewise be a reasonable procedure for weight reduction. By the by, there are different ways to deal with weight reduction for the individuals who would prefer not to tally calories, for example, regimens that attention on dietary conduct changes rather than carbohydrate contents.

Perhaps somebody decides to tally calories or adopt a social change strategy; it is essential to "discover ways to cut calories as well as supplant them with more advantageous decisions that are still sincerely and truly satisfying for that individual."

Somebody intrigued by weight reduction ought to think about how much calories the person is expending, what number of calories the person in question needs, and the contrasts between those numbers. On the off chance that an individual is expending more than anticipated calories, that individual should change their propensity.

It's significant that their conduct change to a "practical example that lessens calories.

Low-calorie slims down

The National Institutes of Health (NIH) states low-calorie slims down as diet plans offer 1,000 to 1,200 calories day by day for ladies and 1,200 to 1,600 calories day by day for men. The number is here and there balanced for activity level, age, and weight. Low-calorie diet designs ordinarily involve customary food, however now and again contain supper substitutions.

"It isn't practical to cut calories. It additionally puts one in danger of losing slender bulk," she said. Individuals, most occasions recover the weight that they lose on low-calorie, consumes fewer calories once they come back to standard caloric admission. "Now and again, they've been keeping to a low-calorie diet for quite a while that they wind up craving unhealthy nourishments or falling into a pigging out example," McDaniel said. The impracticality of low-calorie diets and loss of bulk implies the recaptured weight is regularly fat, not muscle.

At the point when that occurs, said McDaniel, it is doubly hazardous. "In addition to the fact that they were unequipped for continuing something, driving them to feel like they have fizzled, yet then they've likewise deterred the correct proportion between terrible weight [excess fat] and great weight [muscle] and put more [bad weight] on the body framework."

In spite of the fact that McDaniel doesn't prescribe low-calorie diets to be reliably utilized, she says there may be a spot and time for low-calorie feast plans. "The possibility of discontinuous fasting is increasing some prevalence," she said. Discontinuous fasting may involve a day of low-calorie consumption once per week. Irregular fasting stood out after a progression of creature examines demonstrated that it seemed to build a life span. A survey distributed in the diary Cell Metabolism in 2014 found that in people, discontinuous fasting may enable "hypertension, to lessen corpulence, rheumatoid joint pain, and asthma."

"Something like this may be one of the gadgets in somebody's tool stash they can lose for weight reduction," said McDaniel.

Psyche EXERCISES FOR CUTTING CALORIES

Psyche exercise can improve mental wellness, invigorate memory, and lead to a decent time. Similarly, as you practice your body, you have to practice your psyche to keep your cerebrum sharp. Here are ten inventive and fun approaches to utilize your brain:

1. PLAY BOARD GAMES

Playing table games with your friends, friends, and family, families, or associates can be a great deal of fun and keep you thinking quickly. Chess, checkers, imposing business model, act, pictograms, 30 seconds, games, and dominoes can improve your critical thinking abilities, fixation, and general information.

2. LEARN A NEW WORD EVERY DAY

Word-a-day schedules are a simple method to become familiar with other words each day. You can buy into these schedules on the web, buy a physical schedule, or utilize a word reference. This activity will extend your jargon and help.

How to Generate Motivation

Motivation is one of the most potential tools for making lasting change. Your motivation is based on what you believe. And as you probably know, faith is barely grounded in your specific reality. In essence, you create things by how you see them, feel them, listen to them, smell them, etc. You can program your mind by taking emotions from one of your experiences and connecting those emotions with a different experience. Let's see how you can stay motivated to lose weight:

Determine where you are now

You should take a complete picture of yourself in the present as a push mechanism from your current position, as well as for comparison later. Two main factors are related to health. One is if you like the image you see in the mirror and the second is how you feel. Do you have the energy to do what you want and feel strong enough?

Explore the reasons why you want to lose weight. These are the things that will keep you active even when you don't like it.

Assess your eating habits and determine the reasons for overeating or enjoying the wrong foods.

You are supposed to be healthier and lose weight. Here, you clearly and positively declare what you want and then decide that you will achieve it with perseverance. Use the self-hypnosis routine described above to bring this point to your subconscious mind.

Identify your motivation for the desired results and how you will know when you have achieved the goal. How you will feel, what you will see and what you will probably hear when you achieve your goal.

Spend the first self-hypnosis session making the final decision about your weight. Keep in mind that you should not have second thoughts about your weight loss challenge.

Schedule your meals every day. They are often weighed to track their progress as well. However, don't be paranoid about weighing yourself, as this can negatively affect your progress.

Repeat to yourself every day that you are reaching your ideal weight, that you have developed new and sensible eating habits and that you are no longer prone to temptation.

Think positively and give positive confirmations to your hypnotic state.

Adjust your lifestyle

Every little thing counts. This is a crucial thing to keep in mind if you want to lose weight and lose weight. Making a few amendments to your daily activities can help you burn more calories.

Walk more

Take the stairs instead of taking escalator or elevator if you go up or down one or two floors.

Park your car a mile from your target and walk the rest of the way. You can also walk fast to burn more calories.

During the day off, make it more active by taking your dog for a walk in the park.

If you have to travel a few blocks, save gas and avoid walking. For longer distances, dust off the old bike and fly to your destination.

See how and what you eat

A hearty breakfast forces your body to overeat, so you shouldn't miss the first meal of the day.

Brushing after a meal signals your brain that you have finished eating, making you less anxious until the next scheduled meal.

If you need to get food from a restaurant, place your order so you won't be tempted by their other offerings.

Schedule your meals for the week so you can count how many calories you consume in a day.

Eat fast, healthy meals to save time. There are thousands of recipes out there. Do some research.

Eat on a table, not in your car. Conducted foods are almost always fatty and full of unhealthy carbohydrates.

Put more leaves, such as arugula and alfalfa cabbage on your meals, to give it more fiber and make you eat less.

Order the smallest food size if you really need to eat fast food

Start your meal with a vegetable salad. Dip the salad in the sauce instead of tossing.

For a midnight snack, drink from protein bars or just have a glass of skim milk.

Eat before going to the supermarket to avoid the temptation of foods you really don't intend to buy.

Clean your closet by removing foods that will not help you with your fitness goals.

The general idea of these bites is that you need to eat less and move more.

Conclusion

The main reason this guidebook is being written is to help people find weight reduction as easily as possible, and to provide top-down information on how hypnosis works quickly to reduce it. weight.

Many people are confused about choosing or finding a magical counselor, often having no idea how to do it, and here and there, wondering if speculation is warranted, despite all the problems. You should consider the basic standards that go with it when choosing a hypnotic inducer.

Critical rules for choosing a hypnosis practitioner.

You can use the models you need by choosing an attractive professional but be sure to use them. You cannot go wrong with the possibility of receiving them.

1. No fraud. I would rather not manage someone who sells professional business experience. The "no exercise required" and I'll fix it for you. No, you need someone to put the action on the intensity of ecstasy to drive and be an idealist, but to really live.

2. A serious cost. See what the experts in your area charge. His favorite expert is based on being there without time. Why, some charge exorbitant fees, not because they are more talented than others. it's silly and self-critical for these experts. They think they are unique. You may also be tempted to feel this way. Certainly not. Don't just take all the stops.

3. Spend as much time as you need. do a little exploring Think about discovering someone you should trust as a task to accomplish. It could take some time. Talk to professionals on the phone. Take advantage of the free tips. Decipher the comments. You are looking for someone to take on a critical job in your life. Pay attention to this, without bad decisions.

4. You are constantly expected to have a sense of security and respect. In case a magician gives you the creepy, get out. Try not to ignore the warnings about the character. Trance inducers are simple individuals.

5. It has to work. After each meeting, you should feel better, act better, and have more expectations. Again, not charm, but gradual progress. When you don't see progress after a few meetings, quit. Try not to be fooled by such clarifications as: "Your unthinkable soul is preparing for a great change."

"Follow these instructions, and whatever additional standards you have, I'm sure you should do very well.

Hypnosis weighs convincingly on the condensate of exploration behind it. However, it is interesting to see that it is occurring gradually, with enchanting execution through specialist hypnosis specialists and self-hypnosis experts. The more the clinical network and the general population recognize the beneficial effects of hypnosis, the more this common and viable method will be used.

Hypnosis is not just "selective treatment". It is a key part of treatment in general.

Charm is an incredible perk that enhances rapid weight loss, which can make weight loss possible when it's never understood. Also, believe me when I declare that enchanting value is worth all your guesses and regrets.

PART 2

WEIGHT LOSS MEDITATION

Introduction

Do you battle to get more fit? Have you generally pictured yourself as dainty, alluring, and liberated from any wellbeing conditions welcomed on by abundance weight? Do you want to get certain things throughout your life, just to feel kept down by the body that you have?

Now and again, we battle to get more fit since we don't have the correct mentality to do as such. We expect doing physical things like eating well and practicing being everything necessary. An enormous piece of weight reduction is mental. Truth be told, this may be the most significant piece of all. In the event that you don't have a solid outlook and one that is centered around showing signs of improvement, at that point you may battle to really lose the weight. This, yet you may find that you battle since you can't keep the weight off, significantly after you lose it at first.

Weight reduction can be a difficult and overpowering excursion. Many weight reduction assets center generally around your eating routine, which is positively significant however can likewise be overpowering. At the point when you set out on the excursion of weight reduction, you may wind up battling to step away from old propensities that lead to your weight gain in any case. You may end up continually ricocheting to and fro between being "on the cart" and "off the cart," which may prompt you feeling remorseful and battling much more to satisfy your wants of weight reduction.

A weight-loss diet, by definition, requires a reduction in food intake below what the body needs to maintain its current form. There is no real food shortage, but all the built-in mechanisms that ensure our survival record fat loss. This reduction triggers a neural circuit that uses an army of hormones that cause the order of overeating. This mechanism is simply called the famine brain.

Overeating works as the brain's primary reward system for dieting. Unfortunately, researchers have found that weight loss of all kinds uses our neurochemical weapons. If you have too much fat, your body won't know. It only "knows" if you risk losing fat. In a brave attempt to regain homeostasis, our system lowers the hormone levels that signal satiety

155

(leptin and insulin) and pumps the fasting hormone 'ghrelin' into the bloodstream. This hormone results in heightened craving for food leading to extra calorie intake and eventually more weight gain.

Scientists are not yet aware of how the brain and physical starvation system interact to support or override each other. What we know is that many regular diets lead to a mind obsessed with food. Therefore, the root of the problem lies in the brain where this cycle continues.

In this guidebook, we will study self-hypnosis, guided meditation for weight loss, sleep learning system, and different affirmations that can help in reducing weight.

It also covers seemingly ordinary but very influential tricks to get rid of excess fat. We will also learn a few practical habits employing the techniques mentioned above. We will investigate the location of the problem and how it affects us so that we can suggest targeted actions.

Shedding pounds can frequently appear to be overwhelming, particularly in the event that you've stood by too long even to consider beginning the excursion. You won't get results for the time being, and that can be disappointing for a few. Be that as it may, with the utilization of spellbinding, you will have the option to see an adjustment in your negative propensities and self-hurting nourishing way. This contemplation and entrancing will control you through the procedure of tolerance and thankfulness on your excursion to more beneficial and more joyful way of life.

What Is Being Mindful?

The concept of mindfulness was first researched in the 1970s by psychologists and, to this day, it is one of the most intensely studied areas of psychology. Mindfulness is very simply bringing your thoughts back to the present moment so that you are experiencing what is happening in the here-and-now, as opposed to your present moment being colored by apprehensions of the future or concerns over the past.

Mindfulness as a skill is not just a good self-development tool. It can be very helpful in the workplace and even vital in some careers. A centered and sharp focus is vital to jobs like police officers, paramedics, emergency room doctors and firefighters. Being able to maintain focus in the present moment can be a matter of life and death for people in such jobs and certainly for you too, should you be on the receiving end of their services.

It can be helpful in parenting in order to allow us to focus on our children in that moment and enjoy them. Mindfulness can also help us not to project our own fears and desires onto our children, allowing them to simply be who they are and not images of our own making.

Mindfulness can be an excellent tool in studying. Every time you shift your attention to something else, your brain burns glucose to do so. If you are attempting to study without being mindfully present, you will find that you become tired very quickly and struggle to retain the information that you have studied in that session. By being mindful, your brain only has to focus on the task at hand and all your energy can be employed in that task.

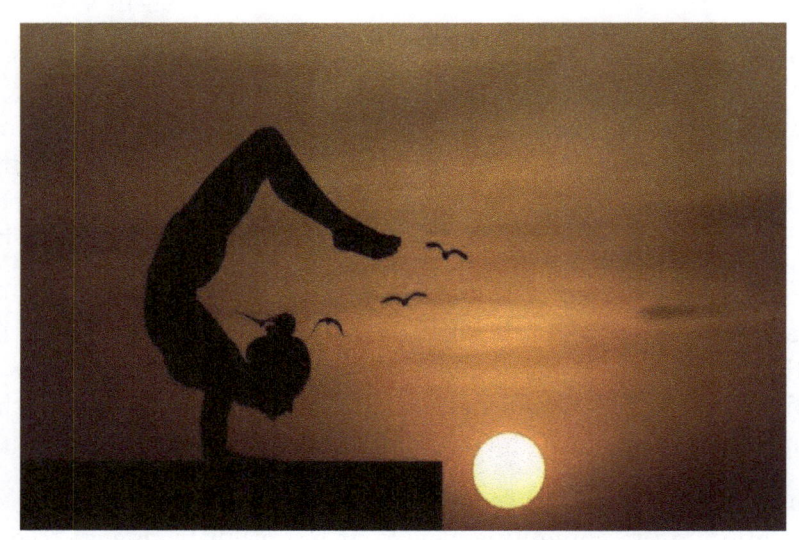

Benefits of Mindfulness for Your Body

One body. That is all you're going to get in this lifetime. That's all everyone is going to get. One life, one body, one mind, heart, and soul. If you don't cherish the body that you have and take care of it the way it deserves, it won't be long before your body starts to break down gradually. You won't even feel it at first or realize that it is happening until it's too late to do anything about it. Your body is the vehicle that you are going to journey through life with, and you must take care of it both on the inside and out for better health physically, emotionally, and mentally.

Mindfulness is one of the many ways in which you will come to realize what your body needs and what it does not, and it certainly does not need the stress that you put it through every day. Actively practicing mindfulness brings awareness to just how much your body is affected by stress, especially when it manifests itself as physical pain. We've covered some of the basic reasons why mindfulness is good for you in general, but now let's focus on what it can do specifically for your body.

Bringing awareness to the way that your body feels through each experience will help you forge a closer connection to your body in a way that you never have before. By frequently "scanning" your body for an overall assessment of how you feel, you start to notice all the little things that you missed before you began practicing mindfulness. You notice every itch, every ache, and every tingle even in the smallest parts of your body. You notice when you start to feel any pain in your body, you notice when you feel cold, warm, pleasantly comfortable, and more. All of the sensations that you feel will always be accompanied by some emotion or thought, and it is through mindfulness that you start to listen to what your body is trying to tell you.

Benefit #1 - Possible Slowdown of Aging Cells. Who wouldn't want to look younger if they could? The beauty industry is a booming business for one simple reason. We're always on the lookout for the proverbial fountain of youth. Anything that holds the promise of turning back the clock and reversing the signs of aging gives us a little bit of hope. Yet, the easiest way to slow down the signs of aging, as it turns out, could be to practice mindfulness to minimize stress. Cell aging is a natural occurrence, but it is sped up by stress, unhealthy lifestyle choices, and the diseases we contract. Some studies suggest that those who practice long-term mindfulness meditation could potentially have greater telomere lengths. Telomeres are a protein that is at the end of the chromosomes in our bodies. This protein is the one responsible for protecting our chromosomes from the signs of aging, and it would seem mindfulness has a positive impact on this. That would explain why some scientists appear to be optimistic that mindfulness could be the anti-aging fountain of youth we've been searching high and low for all along.

Benefit #2 - Better Heart Health. It's no secret that heart disease is one of the leading causes of death, especially in the United States, with one in four deaths annually attributed to this condition. Given that heart disease is associated with chronic stress levels, mindfulness is the way towards better heart health, given the circumstances. In a study that was conducted on participants who were dealing with pre-hypertension, those who learned how to meditate mindfully showed significantly greater improvements in their diastolic and systolic blood pressure levels. This was in comparison to other participants who were given an augmented drug as their treatment instead of a mindfulness program. This suggests that mindfulness could have an important role to play in lowering the risk of high blood pressure and the associated heart conditions that go along with it. Yet another study that was conducted revealed that participants who chose to undergo a mindfulness program had a significant improvement in their 6-minute walking test that measured their cardiovascular capacity.

Benefit #3 - A Healthy Pathway to Weight Management. Weight gain or weight loss are some of the many symptoms associated with excessive stress. Yet, we brush it off and don't think twice about the connection between these symptoms and stress. We don't realize how this behavior pattern and way of thinking of is having damaging effects on our health. When you're preoccupied with stress, there are two ways you could react to it. One, you'll eat in excess as a coping mechanism to feel better, which will result in weight gain. Two, the stress you feel could be so intense that you lose your appetite entirely. Neither approach is healthy, and without mindfulness, it's going to be hard to break out of this destructive cycle. Living in a world today that is designed for convenience certainly isn't helping matters, with fast food and deep-fried unhealthy options available around every corner. The only way to put a stop to it is through mindful awareness. To realize why you feel the way you do, what's causing it, how you're reacting towards it, and what you need to do to put a stop to it.

Benefit #4 - Promotes Better Sleep. It is amazing what a good night's sleep can do for you. Yet, struggling with insomnia and poor, restless sleep at night is becoming an all too common phenomenon these days. Especially when our minds are riddled with worries. How many times have you found yourself lying in bed awake at night, tossing and turning as you tried to get some sleep, yet all you could think about was how stressed you feel? Every day, our lives present us with new challenges. Every day, we try to find a balance between managing our careers, families, relationships, finances, health, and wellbeing. By the time the end of the day approaches, you feel so exhausted, drained of energy that you go through the motions without connecting with the world around you. Excessive worry is going to have both long and short-term effects on your wellbeing. Not getting enough sleep will affect your ability to make decisions, rob you of happiness, and aggravate any physical medical conditions you already have, which are often associated with high levels of stress. You need mindfulness for better sleep at night; it will do your body a world of good.

Benefit #5 - Greater Resilience, Physically and Mentally. Mindfulness is about bettering yourself overall, and it encompasses several aspects that go beyond learning how to control your thoughts. One of these aspects involves building resilience, both mentally and physically, to overcome the obstacles and challenges that are thrown your way. There are only two ways to achieve the goals you set for yourself - one is to set them, two is to achieve them. Most of the time, when we give up and feel physically unable to push forward anymore, it is often because our mind has given up first. Without resilience, the desire to give up can be too overwhelming to reject. Setbacks, failures, disappointments along the way, feeling like every time you take one step forward, you take two steps back, that is enough to wear you down and can diminish the desire that you have to keep on pushing forward. When stress becomes a byproduct of these emotions, your body starts to feel defeated as the symptoms begin manifesting physically in the form of aches, pains, and muscular tension. It won't be long before you eventually give up altogether because it does not seem worth it to keep going anymore.

Benefit #6 - Coping Mechanism for Depression. Depression is one of the most debilitating mental conditions that a person can experience. Depression robs you of joy and makes life feel like it is a constant struggle. Feelings of despair, hopelessness, and unhappiness that cannot be explained threaten to drown you in what may seem to be a never-ending cycle of misery. Some days you don't even feel like you have the energy to get out of bed because depression can be so overwhelming. Sometimes it feels like there is nothing that can help you, and it is exactly why you need mindfulness. It has been used for centuries to achieve mental well-being and happiness, satisfaction, emotional stability. When combined with mindfulness meditation, it reduces and minimizes the risk of experiencing depression by limiting the production of excess cortisol in your body, which has been known to be the cause of many stress-related disorders, depression included. Both mindfulness and meditation are effective in helping you balance the neurotransmitters in your brain, especially dopamine and serotonin, which have been strongly linked to causing depression.

Benefit #7 - It Allows Greater Control Over Your Emotions. Our emotions are sensitive to what is happening around us. When you're stressed, you're emotional. Emotions can get the best of you when you don't know how to control them. This is why learning to slow down your thoughts and emotions deliberately can go a long way towards helping you learn how to exercise greater self-regulation over your actions. Being emotional can make it difficult to keep a clear head, and you react based on your impulses instead. Mindfulness helps you stay in control every step of the way, so you are the one who remains in the driver's seat always.

Benefits of Meditation in Your Daily Life

Building Self-Awareness

For starters let's focus on self-awareness.

Take a minute and honestly ask yourself how aware you are of how your body reacts to specific situations. How do you react to light? How do you react to fear? How do you react to happy events? Take a minute and identify each of these physical manifestations of your mind and evaluate them – why do you react in this way? Have you always acted in the specific manner? What has changed, if anything?

You may notice that as you go through these questions in your mind, other questions and thoughts will enter your mind that you didn't anticipate. This is actually very typical and natural. Often times even if you think that a specific thought or specific trigger will cause your mind to think or work in a specific manner in reality it doesn't necessarily process the information in any specific way. This is why reverse psychology works on certain individuals and backfires on others – not all people react to the same form of stimulus in the exact same manner. Meditation allows you to practice introspection and truly identify how your mind reacts to specific triggers. It's almost as if your mind is doing a mental inventory of how you think, how you process, and most importantly how you react.

Try to think of meditation as a form of mental yoga – here the objective is to forge a stronger link between the mind and body. This is to ensure that your mind is more aware of how your body is responding specifically to cues. Meditation helps us understand our own individual sense of awareness. Helping ground us in the present moment allows us to act and think in a way that keeps us in the present.

Reducing Stress and Anxiety

This is just one benefit –meditation is not intended to enhance one's sense of self simply. In fact, a major reason why so many people get involved in meditation, is because they wish to use the practice to cure themselves of unwanted stress and anxiety that they might be dealing with.

Let's simplify this, shall we?

Why do you think you are invested in meditation?

What do you feel unsure or nervous about starting your meditation program?

Try answering this instead – in the past week what are five negative things that have impacted the way you act, think and react? Make a short list in a separate journal. Have you listed them for yourself? ask yourself how often one of these thoughts has controlled your mind. Let's say you feel unhappy at work – how often have you thought of quitting? A lot?

How often do you think about how badly you want to change jobs? Almost always?

Most importantly how often have you done something that would help you change your job, or extract yourself from that toxic work environment? Odds are you just said never very quietly under your breath. Whether or not you feel like you are ready to admit your thoughts to other people, you yourself know exactly how often you are sometimes even obsessing over the negatives in your life. Do you ever wonder why you don't feel comfortable telling other people how often these negative thoughts come to your mind?

Taking control of the negativity that surrounds you is a key part of ensuring that you lead a healthier and happier life, because this negativity is what breeds stress and causes anxiety to build in your mind. So, if you really want to live a stress free, healthier and most importantly, happier life you are going to want to start by finding a way to reduce your stress levels, and train your mind to focus on productive activities, instead of the anxiety triggers that you have built for yourself.

Honing Mental Clarity

Another common issue many individuals tend to have to deal with is – the lack of clarity that is predominant in today's world. For the most part, research has shown that multiple mental disciplines, such as yoga and meditation, can help control the mind and even improve it. Conditions such as ADHD, which is a form of attention deficiency, have been known to show significant improvement with meditation and meditation-based activities.

While it is common knowledge that physical exercise can help keep the body in shape, what people tend to forget is that the brain needs the exact same thing. Neuro exercises, or mental training activities can potentially keep our brain in shape, and can also weed out certain undesirable mental characteristics, such as depressive thoughts, or anxiety.

One of the fundamental issues currently being studied by scientists is the subject of neuroplasticity. What is neuroplasticity, you may ask? Well, simply put, scientists have begun to discover that, contrary to popular opinion, an individual's brain is not shaped at the time of their birth – in contrast the brain is actually constantly growing and learning, which is why it is possible actually to change our brains to specific forms of mental training. For example, one can retrain the brain to alter or improve multiple personality quirks, such as how attentive you are, how happy you are, how angry you are etc.

Instead of considering emotions such as happiness, or anger, or disappointment individual reactions, think of them as skills. You can train your mind so that you are more skilled at being happy or positive, although odds are you have subconsciously been training your mind to be the exact opposite.

165

Building Focus and Fortitude

However, it is not just mental clarity that is affected by meditation. In fact, a large part of meditation deals with building focus. While the science of the issue has clearly established that meditation can help enhance mental clarity by playing with the neural plasticity of the mind, it also does so on a more chemical level by releasing specific hormones to help counter your stress levels.

When you are stressed out, your body releases certain hormones to let your mind know that it is overloaded. Once your mind starts to register that you are stressed out, the body then starts to release adrenaline because it thinks that your body now needs more energy to help get you through these backlogged tasks. The only problem here is that adrenaline can work against you. While theoretically adrenaline should be helping you to get better and to do your tasks quicker and better. Adrenaline serves an important function in our bodies, but unless we learn to control stress, adrenaline works against us. Instead of helping us get through stressful moments, excessive adrenaline instead increases anxiety, and multiplies our stress reaction.

Keep in mind the release of adrenaline in your body is a physical reaction to fear or danger, or some sort of immediate desperate need – this is a physical reaction, that has been passed on to us from our ancestors, who at the time needed that extra bit of energy to fend off predators or to stay alive.

This of course is where meditation steps in. Meditation gives us a sense of self-worth and power, so that when we are faced with a challenge, we are not immediately dropping the ball and going into "danger" mode – instead we are calmly teaching ourselves to cope, which in turn allows our brain to focus and develop better coping strategies.

Emotional Intelligence

So, what else does meditation help with? Well, for starters, it is also an extremely important tool in the development of emotional intelligence. As you begin to become more aware of your own self and how you react to specific situations, you will also realize that you are attuned to how people around you react to those same situations. This form of awareness is also commonly known as emotional intelligence and is currently considered to be of extremely high value. Indeed, some scientists have begun to prefer the evaluation of emotional intelligence over the evaluation of one intelligence quotient to determine a person's potential.

While you probably ask yourselves multiple times whether or not you are good enough or smart enough, odds are you probably don't ask yourself if you are compassionate enough or if you are a good listener. If you are familiar with the television program, The Big Bang Theory, you've probably seen that the protagonist Sheldon Cooper has been portrayed to be an individual with extremely high IQ, but extraordinarily low EQ factor. In later seasons, this impacts his career growth, as well as his personal life. This is actually extremely common - no matter how smart you are, in order to truly succeed in life, you will find that you will require a certain amount of emotional intelligence.

Start asking yourself the following questions to gauge what your emotional intelligence levels are:

1. Are you generally a calm person? Are you capable of maintaining this calm in stressful situations?

2. Would you consider yourself to be compassionate? Are you well attuned to the needs of others?

3. In your opinion, do you have a tendency to make good decisions?

4. Are you capable of listening to what other people have to say? Do you take people's opinion into consideration?

5. Do you believe that you have a positive influence on the people around you?

6. Are you an impulsive person? How impulsive do you consider yourself to be, on a scale of 1 to 10?

7. What is your standard mind-set – happy or sad?

Were the answers that you just provided generally negative in nature? If so, odds are you have a low EQ, the good news is it doesn't really matter how low your EQ is, because you can actually build on your EQ levels through meditation. The act of meditation not only helps you detach from negative thoughts, it is also known to help you assess and attune yourself to the emotions of other people.

But, most importantly, your emotional intelligence levels will help you deal with years of emotional baggage that have burdened your inner mind control. Gone are the days that you couldn't control your temper. With the help of meditation, you can now actively deal with your anxiety, your depression, and your negative thought patterns, replacing them with solid reasoning skills and problem-solving capabilities.

Relaxing the Mind

And finally, one of the least appreciated and yet possibly one of the most beneficial attributes of meditation – mental relaxation. Think about it...when was the last time you gave your brain a break. Keep in mind that going away on holiday does not count. When was the last time that you sat still for 15 minutes and did absolutely nothing? You didn't mentally list the tasks that you have to do, you didn't make decisions about what you're going to need for dinner. You didn't worry about ten different things that happened today – you literally did nothing.

Why is this important? The more relaxed your brain is the easier it is for you to fall asleep, to manage your stress levels, and to reduce your anxiety. Think of it as your emotional balance, by relaxing your brain you are training it to maintain better emotional equilibrium, which in turn allows you to become a more balanced individual.

How to Practice Mindfulness Meditation

Practicing mindfulness meditation couldn't be any simpler: take a seat, pay close attention to your breath, be in the moment, and when your thoughts start to wander, take a deep breath and pull it back to the present gently. By practicing this regularly, you'll gain a better understanding of your mind and of yourself as well.

The first step to meditating is to find a quiet, clutter-free spot in or around your home. It may be in your room, out in the garden or backyard, or anywhere you prefer, as long as there is little or no distraction. Turn on the lights or sit under natural light.

Setting a specific amount of time for your meditation can be helpful, especially if you're just starting out. For beginners, choosing a short time (anywhere between 5-10 minutes) is ideal. Then, you may gradually work up to an hour or at least 45 minutes each day. Many meditators perform 2 sessions in a day: one is done in the morning upon waking up and one in the evening before bedtime. You may do both or either; the important thing here is to find time, no matter how little, to practice mindfulness meditation.

Taking Your Seat

Having good posture is essential when meditating. Below is a posture practice guide which you can do at the outset of your mindfulness session or anytime you feel the need to. You can do this to stabilize yourself as you find that moment to relax before going out into the chaotic world. If you have any injuries or physical difficulties, feel free modify the steps to suit your specific situation.

Find a good seat: You can sit on anything that gives you a solid, stable seat -- not hanging back or perching. It can be a sturdy chair, a bench, a meditation cushion, a yoga mat on a flat surface, etc.

Pay attention to the position/movement of your legs: If you're using a mat or cushion, sit on it with your legs comfortably crossed in front of you. If you can do a sort of a seated yoga pose, then you may do so. If you're sitting on a chair, position your feet so that the bottoms touch the floor.

Straighten your upper body, without stiffening: Sit up straight yet stay relaxed; do not stiffen your body. Follow the natural curvature of your spine. Allow your shoulders and head to rest comfortably on your vertebrae.

Position your upper arms at your sides, parallel to your body: Let your hands rest on your legs. When your upper arms are positioned properly, your hands will naturally drop to the proper spot. Placing your hands too far forward will actually make your body hunch or bend; too far backwards will stiffen it.

Gently lower your chin and gaze downward: When meditating, it is not really necessary to close your eyes completely, though you may do so. Or, you may stare at anything that appears before you without judging or focusing on it.

Be in the moment and focus on your breath: Relax. Bring all your attention to the various sensations within your body. Follow your breath as you inhale and exhale: focus on the physical sensation as the air moves through your nostrils or mouth, and as your chest or belly rises and falls. Choose a focal point. With every breath, make mental notes such as "breathing out" and "breathing in."

When your attention wanders, gently return: In meditation, it is normal for the mind to wander off, so don't worry if you experience it. What can you do when it does? Simply take a deep breath and pull your focus back to the present. Remember that there is no need to eliminate or block that thinking, simply return gently to your breath and resume meditation.

Pause before doing any physical alterations: If you need to move your body, scratch an itch, or make any other physical adjustments, remember to pause. With intention, move at once and allow a space in between what you feel and what you opt to do.

When your mind starts to wander again: During a mindfulness session, you may find yourself distracted more than once -- and this is normal, too. You will learn to stay more focused and distractions will disappear completely over time. Instead of engaging with or wrestling with distracting thoughts, observe them without the need to react. Simply sit still and pay attention. Then, shift your focus back to your breath without expectation or judgment.

Once you're ready, gently raise your head: Then, slowly open your eyes if you had them closed. Take a few moments. Become mindful of any sounds coming from your surroundings, and of your emotions as well as your thoughts. Pausing for a while, decide how you would like your day to be.

Mindfulness practice may be simple, but it isn't necessarily easy. Always find time to meditate and unearth your inner self. Keep doing the practice and results will eventually accrue.

Other Ways to Practice Mindfulness

More than a form of meditation, mindfulness is also a way of living. Even when you're not "actually" meditating, you can practice mindfulness through the following ways:

Practice mindful eating.

Most of us tend to "eat on autopilot" because we often do it while doing other things like talking, reading, texting, thinking, watching television, or scrolling through webpages or emails. As such, we tend to miss out on the delectable smell and taste of our food. Practice mindful eating by fully engaging with the experience of eating, sans the distractions. Smell your food, touch it, and feel it as you take it in. Be fully present and focus all your attention on what's in front of you.

Take mindful walks.

Walking is another thing we tend to do on autopilot because we do a lot of it every day: it has become an automatic action. To walk mindfully, feel the earth beneath you and focus all your attention to the actual experience. As you walk, notice the movement of your feet and body, as well as your surroundings. Pay close attention as your feet touches and lifts off the ground. Observe what is going on around you. Notice the weather, the sights, and the smells. Feel the world as you travel through it and engage all your senses as you do so.

Take mindful showers.

When you shower, feel the water as it glides across your skin. Notice the smell and texture of the soap, the taste and temperature of the water, the calmness and stillness of you. Listen and watch as the water falls onto your skin and onto the ground. Be mindful of your feelings and thoughts as you do this.

Notice your breathing and body sensations.

Breathing is one of the key practices of mindfulness meditation. Because it is a natural and rhythmic action, it is a good means to bring back our awareness to the present. When you closely observe the way you are breathing, you are also taking yourself into your body and out of your mind. Therefore, you are momentarily freeing yourself from distracting thoughts, fears and worries; basically, reminding yourself of who you truly are – not your thoughts, but your inner spirit.

On the other hand, body sensations like the slight tingling of the muscle or an itch should also be noticed, but without judging or attempting to understand or change them. Simply notice them and then let them go.

Notice your thoughts and emotions.

You are not your thoughts or feelings. The fact that you can observe or notice them means you are separate from and higher than them. Become aware of your feelings, of your emotions, and of your thoughts, but do not judge. Simply observe them as they ebb and flow – like gentle waves in the ocean. Let your attention fall softly on them, without the need to understand or change them. Do not get caught up in them or forget that they aren't who you are. Do not fall into the temptation of getting carried away by your thoughts and emotions into the past or the future. Finally, let them pass away.

Be in the moment.

Be right here, right now: enjoy the present without looking back or far ahead or wishing you were somewhere else. There is no need to worry about a thing because things shall unfold naturally. Let go of any fears and insecurities and concentrate on your present work. Embrace each moment and appreciate the wonders of NOW. Being mindful is also being aware of what's happening at the present moment and doing everything with pure pleasure.

Engage with your senses.

When you're carried away by your emotions, feelings or thoughts, you become disconnected with the HERE and NOW. Your senses – sight, sound, smell, taste, and sound – are your gateway to the present, so do not lose connection with them. Immerse in the delightful aroma of your morning coffee. Revel in coolness of the ocean air, the beauty of trees and flowers in the neighborhood, the gentleness of the sunlight as it hits your skin. Notice the texture of your clothing, and of your bed sheets in the morning. Feel the warmth and passion of your lover's hugs and kisses. Put your attention and love into the simple everyday tasks you do, and you'll be amazed at how much peace and happiness doing so could bring you.

Accept the things you can't change.

Humans tend to wish things were better and hope they could have something they don't have. Nobody seems to be satisfied with their present conditions and with the things that they already have. This would often lead to constant feelings of frustration and discontent. On the other hand, a mindful person does not judge. He accepts things as they are and is able to appreciate their worth fully. Nothing is bad or good – only we create these mental tags.

All of us are blessed with unique, individual powers. By building up your self-confidence and sense of self-worth, and not trying to change the real you, you can be so much more than you've ever thought. Be around people who accept you as you are and who believe in you. Do not try to change everything only because you cannot accept them. Change yourself or other things only for the sake of improvement and learning new things.

Accept your weaknesses.

Nobody is perfect. All of us have imperfections which we must accept. We all make mistakes, and these mistakes are what makes us wiser and stronger. But in order to learn from your mistakes, you must accept and be fully aware of them in the first place. Otherwise, you will fail to recognize your true potential. Instead of feeling defeated by your failure, mindfully analyze the reasons behind it. Pin down your weaknesses and work on them. Do not hesitate to ask help from reliable people if necessary. Asking someone for help will not make you small, but it will definitely make you smarter in the end.

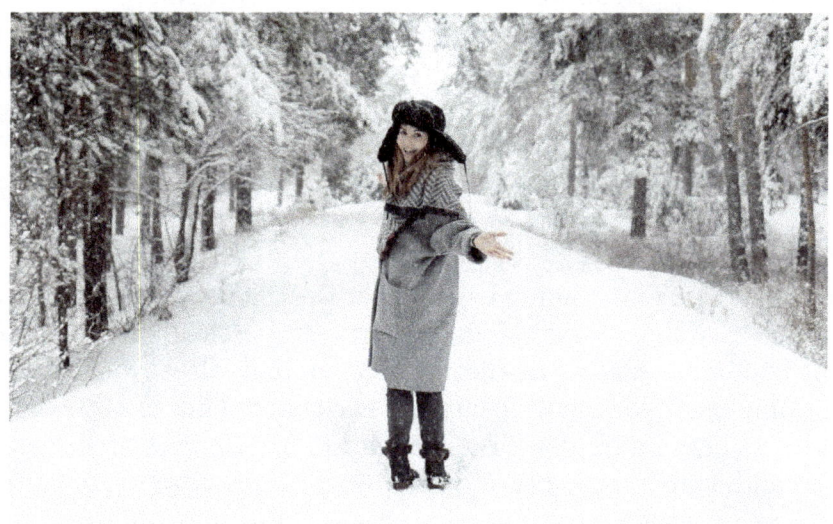

How Can Meditation Help Weight Loss?

You eat what is necessary

At times we eat not because we are hungry but because food is available. The same way you make random decisions to purchase items you don't need in a supermarket in the same way we purchase food at times. For instance, you might recently have acquired a job, and it's your first time to acquire some financial freedom. You find that there is that expensive restaurant you have wanted to go to, but you couldn't afford it since you had money at that particular time. Now that you can afford it to visit it frequently and purchase food that you do not really need but you are buying just because you have the money and food is available. Most of the bad decisions that lead us to eat food that we do not have to eat can be avoided if we focus our thoughts on getting that which is necessary. This process will require that an individual acquires some personal discipline. Before you purchase any food, you ask yourself if it is really necessary. See if the food that you are taking will add any value to your health. After asking yourself such a question, you get to know the right thing to do based on your response to the questions. It is an easy process that will save you from consuming some carbs that make you add unnecessary weight.

Helps us in making the right decisions regarding food

We live in a time where people are becoming creative with food. People are trying out new recipes to see what can work and what cannot. We are having increased production of processed foods as people venture into the food business. At the end of the day, they want to make money and provide foods that people will love and will make them keep coming for more. They learn their target audience and give them what they want. Most people will eat something just because it is sweet, and they like how it tastes in their mouths. You might be hungry, and you are looking for something to eat. You have the decision to choose a healthy meal or eating an unhealthy meal. You know the benefits of taking a nutritious meal, and at the same time, you understand the disadvantages of taking an unhealthy meal. Meditation allows you to make a better and more informed decision regarding your life choices. Some of these life choices are in the decisions we choose to make for the meals that we want to take. Most times, we overlook the power of such decisions and the impact they could have. Meditation allows you to consume that which is necessary at that moment. In this case, you chose to take a vegan meal over some processed food. In the end, you are healthy, and it helps you lose extra weight since you only take foods that are well utilized by your body.

Improves your mode of eating

How do you chew your food? Did you know it can have an influence on your weight? Some of the things we do look simple and you would not expect them to have any effect. Surprisingly, how you chew your food matter. When you chew your food fast and swallow it immediately, the food particles are not well broken down. The body might find it hard to utilize the contents of the food, and much of what you consumed becomes waste. After the food leaves your mouth, it goes through other processes. The body may not be able to break it further, and hence it becomes extra bulk in your body. When this happens, the body converts it into fats, and you end up gaining weight. You might have consumed a little amount of food, but due to your poor mode of eating, you add some extra weight. Meditation allows you to concentrate while chewing food. Once the food particles are completely broken down, it becomes easier for your body to process them. In the process, each nutrient content present in the food consumed is well utilized by the body. Afterward, there will be no extra food that needs to be converted into fats. It prevents you from adding extra weight, and in the process, you get to lose weight.

You realize the effects of certain foods on your body

Once we consume food, our bodies respond to what we have consumed. It could be a negative or positive response. Different foods generate different feelings. We may not believe what some of these feelings are unless we focus our minds on realizing them. The power of meditation is that it allows you to focus, concentrate, and point out certain things that need your attention. This is an easy thing to accomplish; you only need to evaluate how your body reacts to the foods that you consume. After consuming some foods, you will notice that some make you feel energized while some make you feel tired. Anytime you overeat, there is some sudden feeling of tiredness. You feel like your body is too heavy, and all you want to do is take a nap or rest. This is a sign that whatever you ate was unnecessary, and hence the body will not use it. As a result, most of what you ate will be waste that your body needs to eliminate. In that process, you add some extra weight as the excess food becomes excess fat in your body. On the other hand, if you eat and immediately feel energized, it means that your body was receptive to the food that you consumed. It is able to convert much of it into energy, and each component present in the food is well utilized. This is beneficial for the wellbeing of your body and can help you in loss of weight and prevent you from adding unnecessary weight.

It helps you realize your cravings

The various food craving that we have can be caused by a variety of things. You might be busy viewing posts in your various social media accounts, and all over sudden you come across a picture of a good-looking hamburger that seems to taste as good as it looks. Immediately, you develop a need to eat some. Before you saw the picture, such a thought had not crossed your mind, but now that you have seen it, you suddenly want to have some. As a result, you automatically develop a craving for a hamburger. You might find yourself walking to get fast food to get some, or you might want to order some online. The craving makes you make suddenly rushed decisions to eat, which can contribute to adding some extra weight. Some cravings are generated from wanting to consume the foods that we like eating. You might be an individual that loves taking tacos. All you think of any time you want something to eat is how you will get those tacos that you love so much. Being aware of some of these cravings can help you in avoiding them. Meditation helps you to realize the cravings that you have. After conducting an evaluation, you can find out if some of these cravings are beneficial to your body. If you realize that they are doing more harm than good, you get to avoid them.

You get to realize when you need food and when you are full

At times we confuse cravings with hunger. There is a difference between wanting to eat chocolate when you are hungry and wanting to get some food when you are hungry. The chocolate bar contains some sugars that make you full once you consume them. You might be having a busy day at the office, and you grab a lunch bar during lunchtime, and it's probably all that you will eat at that particular time. In that moment of choosing what to eat, you can still decide to eat a healthy meal that will still satisfy the need at that moment. Meditation allows you to distinguish between when you have a craving, and when you are really hungry, this allows you only to eat when necessary. You avoid eating foods that are not helpful to your body, and as a result, you are highly unlikely to gain weight. On the other hand, mediation allows you to know when you are full. Earlier, we stated that we, at times, eat just because food is available and not that we are hungry. With the help of mediation, you can easily know if you are eating food just because it is available or if you for sure need to eat. Such minor decisions are major when it comes to weight loss as they ensure you only eat what your body requires.

You formulate the good eating habits

There are certain ways in which we consume our food. Some of these ways are not beneficial and cause us to create more harm to our bodies. Most of the time, we ignore the time factor as far as eating is concerned. We barely look at the decisions we make regarding food, and all that we do is make some rush decisions. Having an eating routine is very important. Nutritionists are constantly advising us on the right ways to consume our food. For instance, it is wrong to drink water immediately after a meal. You first have to allow the food to settle; then you take your water after some 30 minutes. On the other hand, they advise that fruits should be consumed before meals for them to benefit your body rightfully. When you consume them together with the meals, they may not have the huge impact they would have if; you had consumed them before the meal. Some of these healthy facts are simple and easy to follow; we just choose not to. Additionally, you will find that we consume our foods in moments that we should not be consuming it. For instance, you eat a lot of food at night, and the only activity that you are performing then is sleeping. You find that much of this food is not well utilized in the body, and it becomes waste. The end result is that you end up gaining weight due to poor eating habits. Meditation allows you to realize the impact of the decisions that you make and helps you change how you make decisions. For instance, you may realize that you have poor eating habits and so you decide to change them for the sake of your health and for you to be in the right shape and weight.

Daily Weight Loss Meditation

Before you can begin using meditations to do things such as help you burn fat, you need to make sure that you set yourself up properly for your meditation sessions. Each meditation is going to consist of you entering a deep state of relaxation, following a guided hypnosis, and then awakening yourself out of this state of relaxation. If done properly, you will find yourself experiencing the stages of changed mindset and changed behavior that follows the session.

In order to properly set yourself up for a meditation experience, you need to make sure that you have a quiet space where you can engage in your meditation. You want to be as uninterrupted as possible so that you do not stir awake from your meditation session. Aside from having a quiet space, you should also make sure that you are comfortable in the space that you will be in. For some of the meditations, I will share, you can be lying down or doing this meditation before bed so that the information sinks in as you sleep. For others, you are going to want to be sitting upright, ideally with your legs crossed on the floor, or with your feet planted on the floor as you sit in a chair. Staying in a sitting position, especially during morning meditations, will help you stay awake and increase your motivation. Laying down during these meditations earlier in the day may result in you draining your energy and feeling completely exhausted, rather than motivated. As a result, you may actually work against what you are trying to achieve.

Each of these meditations is going to involve a visualization practice; however, if you find that visualization is generally difficult for you, you can simply listen. The key here is to make sure that you keep as open of a mind as possible so that you can stay receptive to the information coming through these guided meditations.

Aside from all of the above, listening to low music, using a pillow or a small blanket, and dressing in comfortable loose clothing will all help you have better meditations. You want to make sure that you make these experiences the best possible so that you look forward to them and regularly engage in them. As well, the more relaxed and comfortable you are, the more receptive you will be to the information being provided to you within each meditation.

A Simple Daily Weight Loss Meditation

This meditation is an excellent simple meditation for you to use on a daily basis. It is a short meditation that will not take more than about 15 minutes to complete, and it will provide you with excellent motivation to stick to your weight loss regimen every single day. You should schedule time in your morning routine to engage in this simple daily weight loss meditation every single day. You can also complete it periodically throughout the day if you find your motivation dwindling or your mindset regressing. Over time, you should find that using it just once per day is plenty.

Because you are using this meditation in the morning, make sure that you are sitting upright with a straight spine so that you are able to stay engaged and awake throughout the entire meditation. Laying down or getting too comfortable may result in you feeling more tired, rather than more awake, from your meditation. Ideally, this meditation should lead to boosted energy as well as improved fat burning abilities within your body.

The Meditation

Start by gently closing your eyes and drawing your attention to your breath. As you do, I want you to track the next five breaths, gently and intentionally lengthening them to help you relax as deeply as you can. With each breath, breathe into the count of five and out to the count of seven.

Now that you are starting to feel more relaxed, I want you to draw your awareness into your body. First, become aware of your feet. Feel your feet relaxing deeply, as you visualize any stress or worry melting away from your feet. Now, become aware of your legs. Feel any stress or worry melting away from your legs as they begin to relax completely. Next, become aware of your glutes and pelvis, allowing any stress or worry to

181

fade away as they completely relax simply. Now, become aware of your entire torso, allowing any stress or worry to melt away from your torso as it relaxes completely. Next, become aware of your shoulders, arms, hands, and fingers. Allow the stress and worry to melt away from your shoulders, arms, hands, and fingers as they relax completely. Now, let the stress and worry melt away from your neck, head, and face. Feel your neck, head, and face relaxing as any stress or worry melts away completely.

As you deepen into this state of relaxation, take a moment to visualize the space in front of you. Imagine that in front of you, you are standing there looking back at yourself. See every inch of your body as it is right now standing before you, casually, as you simply observe yourself. While you do, see what parts of your body you want to reduce fat in so that you can create a healthier, stronger body for yourself. Visualize the fat in these areas of your body, slowly fading away as you begin to carve out a healthier, leaner, and stronger body underneath. Notice how effortlessly this extra fat melts away as you continue to visualize yourself becoming a healthier and more vivacious version of yourself.

Now, visualize what this healthier, leaner version of yourself would be doing. Visualize yourself going through your typical daily routine, except from the perspective of your healthier self. What would you be eating? When and how would you be exercising? What would you spend your time doing? How do you feel about yourself? How different do you feel when you interact with the people around you, such as your family and your co-workers? What does life feel like when you are a healthier, leaner version of you?

Spend several minutes visualizing how different your life is now that your fat has melted away. Feel how natural it is for you to enjoy these healthier foods, and how easy it is for you to moderate your cravings and indulgences when you choose to treat yourself. Notice how easy it is for you to engage in exercise and how exercise feels enjoyable and like a wonderful hobby, rather than a chore that you have to force yourself to commit to every single day. Feel yourself genuinely enjoying life far more, all because the unhealthy fats that were weighing you down and disrupting your health have faded away. Notice how easy it was for you to get here, and how easy it is for you to continue to maintain your health and wellness as you continue to choose better and better choices for you and your body.

Feel how much you respect your body when you make these healthier choices, and how much you genuinely care about yourself. Notice how each meal and each exercise feels like an act of self-care, rather than a chore you are forcing yourself to engage in. Feel how good it feels to do something for you. For your wellbeing.

When you are ready, take that visualization of yourself and send the image out really far, watching it become nothing more than a spec in your field of awareness. Then, send it out into the ether, trusting that your subconscious mind will hold onto this vision of yourself and work daily on bringing this version of you into your current reality.

Now, awaken back into your body where you sit right now. Feel yourself feeling more motivated, more energized, and more excited about engaging in the activities that are going to improve your health and help you burn your fat. As you prepare to go about your day, hold onto that visualization and those feelings that you had of yourself, and trust that you can have this wonderful experience in your life. You can do it!

Benefits of Meditation for Weight Loss

Below are the incredible ways that meditation can help you achieve daily weight loss:

1. Meditation reduces stress

With meditation, you will feel calmer as well as have a stress-reducing impact on your body. With endless roles in life including work, children, and home activities, it is not surprising that you may be overwhelmed, which may contribute to increased stress. Unfortunately, these stressors affect your body by producing more cortisol, a stress hormone that affects the levels of sugar and insulin in the body. As a result, the hormone causes weight gain. Studies have revealed that meditation activates a relaxation response, regulating the nervous system and, in turn, lowering the cortisol levels.

With a few minutes of deep breathing and conscious relaxation, you will be able to obtain the cortisol-lowering benefits as well as your overall stress levels.

2. Meditation promotes a focus on intention

Often, meditation techniques involve focusing on specific goals or concepts. Meditating on cutting down weight streams your energy, thoughts, and intentions to a particular goal. In this case, you submit to the intentions by revealing your goals to the world, which makes both your conscious and subconscious mind to be aware of the goal that you want to lose some weight. The outspoken intention will stay with you for a long while, enabling you to achieve your weight loss goal both consciously and subconsciously, and dodging all possible distractions.

3. With meditation, you will learn conscious eating

With daily meditation, you will be able to boost your levels of mindfulness and awareness. This can allow you to live in the moment and always focus on what you are doing in the present. The process of meditation can help you gain an increased sense of awareness of actions and thoughts, thus helping you to think twice before you have taken an action. Rather than enabling your cravings to take over you, you will develop the power of controlling your mind, thus handling your cravings with greater intention and awareness. When you are ready to eat, your awareness will make it easier to recognize the textures and flavors of the food you are eating, instead of taking them for granted.

4. Meditation stabilizes mood hormones

Common daily stressors and activities can affect the way your system operates normally and may throw your hormones out of normal functioning. Apart from keeping your cortisol and adrenaline levels regulated, meditation goes further than this. The technique for relaxation releases both oxytocin and serotonin hormones, which boost your moods and ensure your hormones remain stable.

5. Meditation regulates sleep

Lack of sleep may hinder your weight loss progress. You see, by having a deep sleep, your cortisol levels will rise, which in turn will sabotage your progress in losing weight. Also, when you lack sleep, ghrelin, a hunger signal hormone, is also produced in plenty, thereby increasing your chances of eating more for weight gain. With meditation, you will be able to balance the circadian rhythms that promote quality sleep. Meditation increases the levels of melatonin, a hormone that also determines and controls when you sleep.

How to Make Sure that Meditation Works for You

If you want to include meditation in your rapid weight loss hypnosis, it is important that you make it simple. Meditation should help you recover from any stressful event, not become a source of it. That is why you need to consider the three easy ways highlighted below, which you can incorporate in your daily mediation.

Consider a Mantra That Can Help You Lose Weight

A mantra refers to a phrase that one repeats to focus their mind on mediation and bring them to the relaxation state. A mantra can give help you identify something to focus on as you meditate. Although it is very helpful to many people, a mantra is not a must in meditation. You don't need to force yourself to use one if you don't find it helpful or if it does not make you feel natural. However, in case you choose to use one, you need to repeat it as you inhale as well as when you exhale. Some of the common mantras used include "I am at peace with myself," "I am loved," or "I can do this."

Follow Your Breath to Avoid Stress

As you meditate, try to count your inhales 4 ties and exhales 8 times. Remember that meditation is a process that is aimed at reducing stress; if these counts do not feel natural, you should deviate from them. Every time you meditate, always try to increase the number of exhaling and inhaling counts. Do not feel stressed if it takes longer to reach 8 counts. Just keep in mind that lengthening the exhale will greatly affect your health as you will be able to calm down.

Consider a Guided Meditation

If you are not able to practice meditation alone, you should consider a guided process. This includes websites, phone apps, podcasts, and recordings that can help you connect with experts who guide you on how to meditate.

Sitting and Posture

We start by discussing the five basic meditative postures. Your job is to determine which attitude works for you in most situations and stick to it. Although you have to follow a specific meditative posture for certain meditative exercises, most can also be adapted to alternative postures.

Chair Meditation

Since most of us tend to have 9-to-5 jobs, we realistically tend to sit in some office chair for most of our time. Chair meditation is a great way to break through your afternoon monotony without ever having to leave your station. For seated meditation, you want to straighten your back and make sure you hit the floor with your feet. Ideally, your knees should be bent at a 90-degree angle and your back should be as straight as possible. If you're not sure what to do with your hands, just rest them on your knees.

Standing Meditation

Sometimes you want to get out of your chair, and it may be more pleasant to try a standing method. You will want to start standing so that your feet are shoulder-length apart. Bend your knees slightly and relieve pressure throughout your day down to your feet. As you do this, adjust your hands so that they are gently placed over your abdomen so that you can feel every breath moving through your body as you embark on your personal mission.

Kneeling Meditation

If you want to keep your back straight but don't feel comfortable crossing your legs, another great alternative is kneeling. Traditionally this is known as the Virasana or the Vajrasana. Here you start by bending your knees and resting your body weight along the length of your shins. Your ankles should be tucked under your buttocks. For convenience and comfort, you can choose to place a rolled-up yoga mattress or some type of tube between your buttocks and your knees.

This particular position is usually easier than sitting cross-legged and is also generally pain-free, so your ankles will thank you.

Horizontal Meditation

However, if none of these positions suit you, or if you try a sleep-inducing meditation, you will find that the chosen posture is generally the horizontal posture. When laying down, make sure that your feet are shoulder-length, similar to the standing meditation position, and that your arms are at your sides instead of being folded over your body. If you find this position uncomfortable, you can bend your knees and lift your hips slightly to help yourself adjust.

Cross-Legged Meditation

Another pose that you can explore if you feel comfortable is the traditional Indian cross-legged. This particular posture is actually the most recommended posture of meditative activities, the idea being to keep your legs crossed, hips slightly higher than the heels of your feet. If you are new to meditation, it is generally recommended to try this pose with a pillow or towel or some kind of soft surface underneath so that you don't hurt yourself as it can be difficult to hold when that are not used to it. If you feel there is too much pressure on your heels, try bringing one of your legs over the other so that the ankle is one above the knee of the other leg. You can also bring full heels over the thighs of the other leg in what is commonly known as the Lotus position.

The Burmese pose is slightly different because you don't cross your legs. Instead, you can position your feet so that the ankles of each foot are bent inward and facing the pubic area - this pose is generally preferred by people who have a hard time crossing their legs.

Meditation for Fast Weight Loss

Contemplation can be a perception that connects the brain and body to a method for quieting. Individuals have been pondering as a non-mainstream perception for a large number of years. Today, a considerable lot of us are utilizing reflection to decrease pressure and get a great deal of checking out their contemplations. There are numerous sorts of contemplation estimated in a square. The utilization of explicit expressions known as mantras was bolstered by some square measure. Others center around breathing or keeping the brain in the present. Every one of these ways will enable you to build up a vastly improved comprehension of yourself, yet your brain and body cooperate.

This expanded mindfulness makes reflection a helpful device to comprehend your dietary patterns better, which could prompt weight reduction. Peruse on to become familiar with the weight reduction advantages of reflection and how to begin.

What are the advantages of weight loss meditation?

Continued weight reduction

Contemplation won't make you get in shape medium-term. In any case, with a little practice, it might have enduring impacts on your weight, yet additionally on your examples of reasoning. Contemplation is related to an assortment of advantages.

Mindfulness contemplation is, by all accounts, the most accommodating as far as weight reduction. A survey of existing examinations in 2017 found that reflection on cognizance was a compelling method to get in shape and change dietary patterns.

Reflection of care includes giving close consideration to where are you, and are you doing what you feel right now? All through the contemplation of care, you will perceive every one of these perspectives without judgment. Attempt to regard your contemplations and activities as those by themselves—nothing else. Consider what you feel and do, yet don't attempt to group anything as positive or negative. Standard practice makes this simpler.

189

Rehearsing reflection with mindfulness can likewise bring about long-term benefits. As per a 2017 survey, the individuals who practice mindfulness are bound to keep the weight off contrasted with different health food nuts.

Less blame and disgrace

Contemplation of care can be particularly helpful in checking passionate and stress-related eating. You can perceive those occasions when you eat because you are pushed, instead of hungry, by ending up progressively mindful of your considerations and feelings.

It is additionally a decent instrument to keep you from falling into the unsafe winding of disgrace and blame for which a few people fall when they attempt to change their dietary patterns. Contemplation caution includes recognizing your sentiments and practices for what they are, without deciding for you.

How might I start to mull overweight reduction? Reflection can be polished by anybody with the psyche and body. No extraordinary gear or costly classes are required. For some, finding the time is the hardest part. Attempt to begin with a sensible thing, similar to 10 minutes per day or even every other day.

Ensure that during these 10 minutes, you approach a tranquil spot. You might need to crush it in on the off chance that you have children before they wake up or after they hit the sack to limit diversion. In the shower, you can even attempt to do it.

Make yourself agreeable once you are in a tranquil spot. In any position that feels simple, you can sit or rest. Start by concentrating on your breath, watching the ascent and fall of your chest or stomach. Feel the air moving all through your nose or mouth. Hear the sounds that the air makes. Do these for a couple of minutes until you feel increasingly loose?

Please follow these steps with your eyes open or shut:

- Take a full breath in.

- Keep it for a couple of moments.

190

- Exhale gradually and rehash.

Breathe.

- Observe your breath as it streams into your noses, raises your chest, or moves your midsection, however not the slightest bit modify it.

- Continue centering for 5 to 10 minutes on your breath.

- You're going to discover your mind, meandering, which is very ordinary. Simply perceive that your psyche has meandered and taken your consideration back to your breath.

- Reflect on how effectively your brain meandered as you wrap up. Perceive then that it was so natural to reestablish your regard for your breath.

Attempt to accomplish a larger number of weekdays than not. Remember that in an initial couple of times you do, it may not feel exceptionally effective. Be that as it may, it will end up less complex with successive exercise and start to feel progressively regular.

The Power of Repeated Words and Thoughts

Recollect how you used to rehash something again and again so as to retain it for a test? At the point when done over some stretch of time, rehashed words and contemplations will in general become lasting. By rehashing your insistences, your brain will gradually surrender and Believe what you're letting yourself know.

Reinventing the Subconscious Mind

The psyche mind is the most remarkable piece of our cerebrum, but at the same time it's the hardest to control. Inside the inner mind, the entirety of your actual expectations, dreams, fears, and bad dreams are put away.

The motivation behind why a few insistences don't work is that the psyche mind has not been persuaded and is consequently as yet pulling in negative occasions. All together for your insistences to begin producing results throughout your life, you need to fool the inner mind into tolerating your certifications.

Here are a few hints to enable your confirmations to break through to your inner mind:

Discover the harmony among aspiring and reasonable – many individuals go over the edge with their confirmations. A few people who are gaining next to no and are covered in the red may attempt to state, "I am rich, and I win $100,000 every month." obviously, the inner mind knows immediately this isn't accurate. One approach to fix this isn't really to mitigate the fantasy, yet to include more authenticity into it, e.g., "I have the quality and assurance to liberate myself from obligations and work harder to procure $100,000 every month."

Give your inner mind confirmation that your assertions are valid – insistence alone won't transform you; you need to blend in real life also. Confirmations like "I have a strong constitution" are pointless if not joined with appropriate exercise, rest, and sustenance. A superior variant of the past insistence would be: "I decide to practice in any event three times each week, get at any rate 7 hours of rest, and eat well food in light of the fact that my strong physical make-up is on its way."

Make certifications that inspire forceful feelings – notice how many individuals recall effectively occasions that made them cry, chuckle, and so on. Ensure that when you make confirmations, you incorporate descriptive words that bring out cheerful, moving and inspirational considerations. Rather than saying "I decide to get up early every morning," state, "I decide to get up early every early daytime feeling energized, revived, and prepared to take on the day!"

Ensure your assertion targets you – tailor your insistences particularly for yourself. For instance, an attestation like "My supervisor will give me an advancement" is somewhat frail since that assertion focuses on your chief and not yourself; you don't have any power over your chief. Rather, settle on something like "I decide to feel that I generally get quality work turned in and thusly merit an advancement."

Guided Meditation for Weight Loss Sessions

We tend to turn to food whenever we are stressed in life. When problems overwhelm us, most of us tend to stress-eat, and then we experience a cycle of guilt and regret. In time, this cycle can impact how we feel about ourselves.

During this guided meditation, you will remember how to feel good and understand your connection to food. During times of stress, you will learn about letting go of tension and to experience all that is natural and instinctive.

The experience of this guided meditation will be enhanced if you find yourself a comfortable and ventilated spot.

Ensure that there is no disturbance from anything or anyone for thirty minutes.

You need to choose a position to lie down or maybe sit comfortably for the duration of this exercise. It is a good idea at this time to unplug or mute your phone.

Now, you need to close your eyes and prepare for a deep sense of relaxation and wellbeing. Remember that this is your time, and embrace the opportunity to escape from the stressful world you live in. You can now relinquish all the unhealthy habits and learn to boost your inner spirit.

With your eyes closes, breathe deeply and slowly through your nose and then exhale through your mouth. When you breathe in, you are taking all that is good and positive about this world into your body, and when you breathe, you are letting go of all tensions and unnecessary fears.

Now, inhale again. Breathe in slowly through your nose to the count of four.

When you breathe in, you can slowly feel your diaphragm expand when you feel the air enter your lungs. Breathe in until you feel like your lungs are full of air.

Strive to control the exhalation of air and make sure that you breathe out steadily

You need to continue this cycle of rhythmic breathing.

Inhale to the count for four.

Hold your breath for a count of two.

Exhale your breath to the count of four.

You can resume breathing normally, and you will feel all the tension in your body slowly dissipate.

Acknowledge that your body is now starting to feel more relaxed. Your arms and legs will start to feel heavier.

Relax the tension in your lower back, middle-back and your upper back. We often tend to store tension in our shoulders. Learn to release it. When you let go of the tension you feel in your body, you can feel your body relax.

Elongate your neck so that there is space between your ears and shoulders. When you slowly elongate your neck, you can feel the mattress you are lying on or the chair that you are sitting on support your back.

Now, scan your body and check if there are any areas of tension left. If you feel that there are some, then you need to tighten the muscles in those areas and let go deliberately. Once you do this, you can feel your body relax. You can feel the tension leaving your body.

Now, you need to go into a state of deep meditation.

To do this, you need to continue the rhythmic breathing exercise.

Imagine that you are now standing in a beautiful meadow with soft rays of sunlight falling on you.

You can see an arched doorway that is carved into a rising cliff.

Your surroundings look quite peaceful and you feel good.

You can see golden sandy beaches behind you and azure blue skies above you.

Now, you are slowly making your way to the arched doorway. The door is within your reach; the wood feels warm under your fingers. As you trail your fingers across the door, you can feel a sense of excitement and wonder as you imagine what lies behind the door.

To enter, you need to keep your mind open to the wonders that lie ahead. Reach out and slowly turn the handle of the door.

As you emerge, you can see a lush and beautiful, bright-green rainforest.

The air feels cool and pleasant under the canopy and the welcome change from the sun-drenched beach a few moments ago.

Take a deep breath and then exhale to embrace this sense of peace.

As you start to walk forward, you notice a trail that leads through this beautiful rainforest.

As you look up, you can see the glimpses of a beautiful blue sky that's speckled with soft, cotton-like clouds.

Continue scanning the sky all around you.

You are surrounded by majestic mahogany trees that reach up tall towards the zenith.

You marvel at the dark brown bark of the trees that seems to have a very pleasant sweet odor.

Space is limited here, but you are grateful for the narrow trail that leads you through this place of natural wonder.

You can listen to the melodious chirping of birds all around you.

It feels like the forest has come alive around you.

All of this appeal to your senses and you are able to experience nature in its pristine form.

Consider if you strip back your own life and were to live more naturally, how much better you will feel.

Only a small percent of sunlight can penetrate onto the floor of this rainforest. So, you move further out in the wilderness, you can see the flashes of exotic blue butterflies dancing around you.

You can hear the melodic sound of running water in the distance and you feel compelled to move towards it.

As you take in the wonder of the beautiful nature all around you, you move towards the larger expanse of the forest area that leads to a delicate stream of water.

There are natural stepping-stones that lead you to a pool of water that looks crystal clear. The pool of water is surrounded by green plants.

You walk closer to the pool and you notice plants with colorful berries all around.

There are several fruit-bearing plants, and everything looks rich, exotic and absolutely tempting.

You take a bite of these delicious berries and you can feel a burst of flavors.

The berries taste delicious, and you can feel this deliciousness as it makes its way down to your stomach.

Your body feels energized.

There are stones that are present around and across the water and as you walk, you start to become one with nature.

You notice carefully carved out steps higher in the rocks and you start to climb.

The climb is quite easy, and it feels almost effortless.

You feel a wonderful stretching in your muscles when you grip the rocks for balance.

There is no fear of falling.

As you grip the rocks and make your way up, you feel slimmer, stronger and toned.

You feel exactly how you want to feel and how you want to be.

You pull yourself up higher and higher. You are slowly progressing towards the canopy.

You can feel the air become purer.

You start to breathe in pure oxygen and let go of any tensions you are holding onto.

Your 'normal' seems like it is miles away.

You consider how good you feel at this moment.

You continue to make your way towards the canopy.

You don't have to fear the height since it is safe, and you cannot fall.

You don't feel tired or exhausted. In this world, you feel fit, healthy and experience an abundance of energy. You are determined to get to the top and see the view from the top of the canopy.

Imagine walking up through all these steps until you reach the final step and you reach the pinnacle of your journey.

You reach a large platform that overlooks the tops of the trees.

Directly across from you there is a rock face with water cascading down. The water is frothing up on its way down the rocks and the sight is mesmerizing.

You can reach up and touch the clouds. You can feel the clouds around you.

The sky looks beautiful.

Visualize all these wonderful sensations that course through your body in this instance.

You experience a sense of relaxation. Every inch of your being feels good.

Take this moment and visualize yourself stretching.

Keep your arms behind your head and your elbows wired. Engage your core muscles and try to lift your shoulder and your head up towards the clouds up above.

Visualize yourself lifting and engaging those core muscles while you draw in your stomach and tighten your abdomen. All of this makes you feel so good.

Now start to relax once again.

Start to concentrate on your breathing. Inhale as you open up your chest and exhale slowly.

It is time that you start to feel good about the person you are. It is time to feel content and embrace pure inner peace. Here in this rainforest, you are free to explore and be the person that you want to be.

Let go of any unhealthy eating habits, it is time to be kind to your body and to nurture and protect your body.

Repeat these affirmations to yourself and believe in each word.

Believe in the message and the power these words have to change your life.

I will change my perception of my body.

I recognize my self-worth.

I will change my eating habits so that I see my food as fuel and nutrients rather than comfort food.

I will exchange binge eating for breathing techniques and guided visualization.

I will start exercising and changing how I look and feel.

I will create an activity diary and plan how to embrace exercise.

I am ready to face my inner fears and make the necessary positive changes.

Sit quietly for a moment and let these affirmations become a part of you.

It is time to feel positive about your life.

It is time to face any weight issues head-on.

You have the power to do so.

At any time, you can return to this rainforest and experience the wonders of nature. You can find your inner strength and inspiration in this safe haven.

You are centered, and you retain the feeling of peace and wonder.

Enjoy the moment and the feeling of harmony that you experience.

Breathe in and then out.

Retain your sense of peace and your desire to nurture your body.

Breathe in and out.

You will change your association with food.

Breathe in and out.

Slowly open your eyes on the count of three.

One, two and three.

Now, you are back in your reality.

Stretch your body slowly and continue to take deep breaths.

Realize how good you feel in this moment.

Remember your desire to improve your fitness and your wellbeing.

Return to this safe haven of yours whenever you want to improve your health.

You can use this technique anytime you feel tensed or nervous. Whenever you feel stressed, instead of reaching for a packet of chips or any other junk food, you can try this simple exercise to calm your mind. You can literally breathe your way to a stress-free life.

How to Use Meditation and Affirmations?

Have you attempted and neglected to get in shape? Assuming this is the case, you realize how troublesome it very well may be to stay with a weight loss program. What's more, in any event, when you do figure out how to drop those additional pounds, keeping them off is another fight together. In any case, you don't need to spend a mind-blowing remainder doing combating with your willpower with an end goal to get and stay thin.

One of the key contrasts between those individuals who figure out how to get more fit and keep it off effectively, and the individuals who don't, is that the previous gathering changes their eating and exercise propensities as well as their mindset also. If your mind isn't your ally, getting more fit will be troublesome or inconceivable because you'll be continually undermining your endeavors. How about we investigate what's required for the sort of mindset that prompts lasting, sound weight loss.

Persistence

Right off the bat, you should show restraint. The individuals who shed pounds gradually and consistently are well on the way to keep it off. So, overlook each one of those diet designs that guarantee you can shed 10 pounds or more in seven days - the vast majority of that will be water weight, and will be recovered right when you begin eating ordinarily. It's just human to need a convenient solution; however, if you need to lose the weight, keep it off and move on without having to battle with your body for an incredible remainder continually, it merits adopting the moderate strategy, since compromising makes weight loss increasingly troublesome and tedious over the long haul.

Adaptability

Adaptability is likewise significant for effective long-haul weight loss. If you make amazingly inflexible guidelines about what you can and can't eat, you may get more fit, yet risks are you'll be hopeless. You're probably not going to adhere to those principles for an incredible remainder. What's more, when you have this 'win or bust' sort of mindset, and you disrupt your guidelines even somewhat, it very well may be enticing to go on a hard and fast binge a short time later, because all things considered, you've blitz now! Then again, if you follow reasonable rules while recognizing that there will be times, (for example, occasions and unique events) when you'll eat food that isn't a piece of your ordinary diet, at that point these 'illegal nourishments' will appear to be less appealing because they're not something that you've restricted from your life forever.

Consistency

Consistency is another piece of a fruitful weight loss mindset. This may appear to repudiate the above point. However, it doesn't generally. Interestingly, you eat strongly and follow your activity plan most of the time. Along these lines, you'll stay away from yo-yo and unfortunate practices, for example, the binge/starve cycle. It's the moves you make most of the time that will give you the outcomes you are looking for. When you're focused on making long haul changes in your way of life, instead of searching for a convenient solution, you'll be increasingly spurred to embrace a moderate and adjusted arrangement that you can try reliably.

Self-Love

It is additionally imperative to have an inspirational mentality towards yourself. Presently in case you're similar to a great many people who need to shed pounds, odds are you don't feel generally excellent about your body and appearance. While you don't need to claim to cherish something that you loathe about yourself, it's likewise significant not to be continually beating yourself up for not being at your objective weight as of now. In case you're one of the numerous individuals who will, in general, overheat because of stress, such self-recriminations will most likely cause you to feel even unhappier and significantly increasingly inclined to overeating - thus the endless loop deteriorates.

So, put forth an attempt to concentrate on those things you do like about yourself, and if you have days where you miss exercises or don't eat just as you'd like, be mindful so as not to blame yourself too brutally. Rather, recognize this is something that happens to everyone, and give a valiant effort to put it behind you and start anew simply. Recall that you don't need to eat or practice flawlessly to shed pounds - you simply need a moderate system that is sufficient.

If you can make these things part of your ordinary mindset, weight loss ought to be simpler. It tends to be fairly testing, particularly in case you're accustomed to having a negative disposition towards yourself and your weight loss endeavors. One thing that can assist you with adopting a progressively empowered mindset all the more effective is to utilize a weight loss meditation recording. If you utilize a quality chronicle that incorporates brainwave entrainment innovation, you can increase simpler access to your subconscious mind and utilize basic procedures, for example, affirmations and perception to reconstruct it with new convictions that work for you as opposed to against you.

Such accounts contain dreary hints of explicit frequencies, which make it simpler for your brain to enter a deeply loose and centered state. In such express, the subconscious is increasingly open to the proposal, and any affirmation or perception work that you do will be progressively successful. This is an extraordinary method to assist with changing your mindset from the back to front, regardless of whether you're not knowledgeable about meditation or other mind control procedures. It's justified even despite the little exertion that it takes to do this, since rolling out positive improvements throughout your life, for example, getting more fit is such a lot simpler when you have your mind on your side. You don't have to depend on willpower to battle your self-dangerous inclinations - because those desires aren't there anymore.

Positive Affirmations for Weight Loss Sessions

Tune in and repeat (mentally or softly) the following positive affirmations.

Do it every day for 21 days. Ideally after finishing a meditation because your subconscious will be more receptive.

For whatever length of time that you repeat the affirmations, strive to smile and feel the sentences vibrate inside your heart.

LET'S BEGIN:

I am sound

The universe favors me with wellbeing

I have a solid body

I am grateful for a solid body

Wellbeing Comes to Me

I tune in to my body with affection

It is anything but difficult to settle on sound decisions

I am encircled by a solid way of life

I settle on decisions to improve my wellbeing consistently

I have vitality

I eat food that is supporting and bravo

I have smart dieting propensities

My body recuperates rapidly and without any problem

I am fit as a fiddle

I feel better

All that I do prompts a solid way of life

I am upbeat that I am sound

I am cheerful

I am carrying on with a long and solid life

With Gratitude I deal with my body

I am appreciative for wellbeing

I have life

My body is wonderful simply the manner in which it is.

I love myself and my body.

I am sure and alright with my body.

I am thankful for my body's capacity and quality.

I grasp the shrewdness of my body.

I look and feel energetic.

I am thankful for acceptable wellbeing at each age.

Source is coursing through me.

I am energized and upbeat at the present time.

I adjust my expectations to the vitality of the Universe.

I discover vitality in intentional work.

I emanate positive vitality and imperativeness

Consistently is loaded up with delight and great wellbeing.

I am eager to begin the day.

I draw in wellbeing

Wellbeing is pulled into me

My solid body can rapidly recoup and recuperate

I am grateful for my wellbeing

Eating well prompts a solid body

I am honored with wellbeing

My appreciation for wellbeing brings more wellbeing

I have a sound soul, psyche and body.

My thankful heart pulls in wellbeing into my life

Flawless prosperity is my steady state

I think solid contemplations

I draw in a sound life

My body is sound all around

It is my decision to be sound

I am loaded with appreciation

Wellbeing is my bequest

I experience flawless wellbeing

I have quality

Exercise and eating right are incredible approaches to remain sound

I put stock in my capacity to cherish and acknowledge myself for who I am.

I set myself liberated from all the blame I heft around the food I picked previously.

Consistently I am practicing and dealing with my body.

Mending is occurring in both my body and brain.

Each time I breathe in, new vitality fills my general existence and each time I breathe out, all poisons and muscle versus fat leave my body.

My wellbeing is improving increasingly more consistently, as is my body.

All that I eat mends and feeds my body, which causes me to arrive at the perfect weight.

I am consistently nearer to my optimal load with every single day.

I can do this, I am doing this, my body is getting in shape at this moment.

I am relinquishing any blame I hold around food.

Eating well nourishments enables my body to get the entirety of the supplements it should be fit as a fiddle.

I feel my craving for fat-rich nourishments dissolving.

I have a compelling impulse to eat just sound nourishments and let go of any handled food sources.

I totally comprehend that unfortunate nourishments don't assist me with getting more fit, so I eat just solid, nutritious nourishments.

I love eating well nourishments.

How to Practice Every Day?

At this point, you've presumably taken a stab at everything to shed off those annoying pounds, from confining your calories to intensifying your exercise schedule. While these endeavors may be helping you shed a pound or two at regular intervals, there's something that can give you that additional lift: meditation.

This without cost, normal, straightforward system can be exceptionally powerful in helping you thin down, while likewise mitigating pressure and tension. The exploration encompassing careful meditation rehearses proposes that meditation is firmly connected to weight loss.

The ideas of care and meditation cannot just lower your feelings of anxiety and lift mindfulness. Having a mindful psyche can keep you from overeating and enthusiastic eating. Because of this, meditation for weight loss can be a powerful approach to get in shape and eat better.

Meditation is the demonstration of concentrating on getting progressively careful. As indicated by the American Meditation Society, during meditation, an individual's consideration streams inwards as opposed to taking part in the external universe of movement. The training includes freeing the psyche with the point of coming back to a condition of quiet feelings and clear reasoning.

A few people practice meditation for just five minutes per day, however, specialists recommending attempting to stir that up to around 20 minutes per day. For those who're simply beginning, consider taking five minutes soon after you wake up to clear your psyche before continuing ahead with your day.

Close your eyes and just spotlight on your breathing example without attempting to transform it. If your psyche meanders, which is very basic when beginning, simply control it back to your relaxing.

Expectation and Motivation

The principle motivation behind why meditation can be so powerful in helping individuals get thinner is that it adjusts the cognizant and the oblivious brain into concurring on the progressions that you need to apply to your practices. These progressions incorporate controlling yearnings for undesirable nourishments, changing dietary patterns, and finding the inspiration to work out.

It's therefore essential to have the psyche associated with your weight loss venture because it's the place the destructive, weight-picking up propensities including enthusiastic eating are settled in. Meditation in a perfect world encourages you to become progressively mindful of these propensities and musings, conquer them with time, and even supplant them with positive, solid propensities.

Building up a meditation routine will likewise assist you with keeping weight loss alive. It carries the item to the cutting edge of your brain and your day. Along these lines, it's a lot harder to overlook, which will propel you to continue onward.

Meditation makes a more significant level of fixation and spotlights on your weight loss objectives. Since it's so natural to get occupied, removing some time from your bustling day to ponder will harbor that inspiration.

Mental Well-Being

Meditation and care have additionally been appeared to improve mental wellbeing. Care has been appeared to bring down enthusiastic eating, gorging, and by and large improve the weight loss process.

Stress alleviation is probably the quickest advantage of meditation. It removes you from the battle or-flight mode by bringing down the degrees of stress hormones in your body. Stress hormones, for example, cortisol generally signal the body to store more calories as fat. Because of this, high cortisol levels are going to make it much difficult for you to shed additional weight, regardless of whether you're reliably settling on solid decisions.

As per an examination led via Carnegie Mellon University, everything necessary is around 25 minutes of meditation three days straight to lessen pressure significantly. In another 2016 investigation, members indicated expanded unwinding, consideration, mind-body mindfulness, serenity, and even cerebrum action in the wake of finishing a couple of short meditation sessions. The investigation additionally expressed that degrees of restraint could increment with day by day meditation practice.

At last, in an ongoing exploration survey, specialists assessed that the job of meditation on weight loss, alongside the practices that are often connected with poor eating. They presumed that careful meditation could be useful in diminishing the recurrence of gorging and passionate eating.

Care

Even though care is very different from meditation, the two ideas go connected at the hip. Meditation causes you to let go of things to come and past. Maybe you have had various bombed endeavors at weight loss previously or you're encountering a few tensions about the future, for example, disposing of poor propensities. Care while reflecting lets you appreciate the present without focusing a lot on these stressors.

Instructions to Ensure that Meditation for Weight Loss Works for You

-       Pick the Right Practice

There are various meditation styles that you can go with, however, they all follow a comparative essential method of quieting the brain and setting aside some effort to inhale and getting mindful of the present minute. It's astute to attempt various techniques that sound fascinating to you to discover which ones work best.

-       Think about Aromatherapy

Fragrance based treatment has additionally been demonstrated powerful in quieting the body, which is useful when meditating. You can by and large use fragrance-based treatment for meditation in two different manners. The first is diffusing the oil into the air.

This can be useful in advancing unwinding, invigorating the faculties, and making an encompassing space where you can truly center. Then again, have a go at utilizing fundamental oils in an individual fragrance-based treatment diffuser like Zen, Vibrant, Active, or Healthy MONQ. Delicately inhale MONQ into your mouth and afterward out through your nose. MONQ ought not to be breathed into the lungs.

Furthermore, fundamental oils can be applied topically to the skin after weakening with a bearer oil.

- Sharpen the Practice

There are additional books that show you how to ruminate. The individuals who are new to the idea of meditation can especially profit from these. If you'd be intrigued to attempt meditation in a guided gathering setting, consider evaluating your nearby meditation community. Most towns and urban focuses have offices or schools where meditators of different levels meet up to rehearse.

Care and Meditation in real life

Meditation and care are known to improve mental wellbeing. Care has been appeared to bring down passionate eating, overeating, and by and large upgrading weight loss.

Constant pressure is related to a more noteworthy grouping of fats in the mid-region, particularly through the overproduction of the pressure hormone cortisol, which is additionally connected to higher mortality. Because of this connection, an examination from the University of California at San Francisco concentrated on identifying in the case of bringing down feelings of anxiety through meditation can help bring down the convergence of tummy fat.

The examination was distributed in 2011 in the Journal of Obesity and explored a gathering of 47 hefty or overweight female members (with a normal of 31.2 bodies mass record), giving a portion of them a progression of classes about care meditation systems.

The classes included instructing them on the best way to focus on impressions of nourishment longings, hunger, identify enthusiastic eating triggers, learn self-acknowledgment, and become mindful of negative feelings. The guided meditations were given to present new careful eating abilities, for example, giving a nearby consideration to the flavor of nourishment just as eating more gradually than expected.

All in all, the examination bunch got nine classes, each enduring more than two hours, alongside a quiet retreat day where they were urged to rehearse their new careful eating and meditation abilities. They were additionally urged to utilize the careful abilities when they returned home in assignments of as long as 30 minutes out of every day during or before dinners, six days per week, and to sign in their meditation action.

Both the benchmark groups and the examination bunch got additionally got a two-hour nourishment and exercise data session. Toward the finish of the exploration time frame, the entirety of the members was estimated for their circulation and measure of stomach fat, alongside their cortisol levels.

Two key results of the examination were assessed: regardless of whether the pressure decrease, and careful eating program diminished passionate eating and whether it influenced the measure of paunch fat in members.

As a rule, the investigation found these rehearsed diminished passionate eating, decreased feelings of anxiety, expanded consciousness of their real sensations, and diminished nourishment yearnings.

Moreover, blood cortisol levels were lower in the treatment bunch contrasted with the benchmark group. Additionally, members who encountered the most significant upgrades in their careful eating, commonly, had a more prominent familiarity with their craving sensations, that were increasingly fruitful at lessening their incessant pressure and encountered the best decrease in stomach fat.

If you are tired of quitting, and you seriously want to do something about yourself, then you know that you are setting yourself on a journey that has its course. Using hypnosis to influence you're eating habits needs a great deal of willpower, and the initial key to move from the dead point is to take some action. The best way to transform your lifestyle successfully and build healthier eating habits is to make a good and detailed plan.

First of all, if you decide to use hypnosis to help you change your perspective about food and you don't want to go to the hypnotherapists, don't worry, there are a lot of links and online resources that offer information, coaching, and sessions. After you determined what kind of sessions you want, the next step is to choose the food and exercise tracking system that you will use to be aware of the real situation.

You can track your food intake manually or through an app. The thing is you need to put down every item and see what works and what you need to change. Daily calorie intake is something that you need to adjust from day to day, and there are calculators made just for that purpose.

After you went through all these details, you need to be prepared to track your weight. Don't forget that the scale is your best friend in this process because it will show you the truth. If you think that you can replace poor food choices with the better ones without some physical activity, think twice. You can burn a few meals with calories through simple exercises. Make your exercising schedule and stick to it.

Thinking through your meals and snacks for the week will keep you from unnecessary overeating. To make sure that your food keeps up with your budget and your lifestyle, plan a shopping list. You should also consider making eat-out options in case you need to go to a business lunch, or you were just invited to a party. This kind of planning helps you to prepare your environment. If you already know what you'll eat, you will bypass your trigger foods, and you'll keep yourself on track.

Being surrounded by people who support you is important for your weight management. You need to put yourself first and try to enroll your family and friends. In the end, make sure you plan enough time for your daily hypnosis sessions and meditations.

Love your Body and Soul

You look in the mirror and you are dissatisfied. Do you wish that your shape, your nose, your legs, your hair were like somebody else's? Why do we always compare ourselves? Why aren't we reconciled with our appearance? We have heard ad nauseam that we should love ourselves, despite our mistakes or flaws. This includes things related to our personality as well as our bodies. However, there are very few people who can accept and be content with themselves. It is not about not wanting to change. It is a commendable endeavor when one wants to achieve or retain their looks or care about looking more attractive.

At the same time, most people are much more critical, stricter with themselves than justified. They are continuously dissatisfied with themselves and don't see in the mirror what others see. Some girls feel a significant discomfort looking at each other, both because they don't like looking at each other in general, and because they don't like what they see. Where do these reactions come from?

What usually happens is that you don't look at yourself; you only see yourself with respect to that ideal of beauty that you have in your head. This is where dissatisfaction creeps in. It has to do with the theory of social confrontation. We compare ourselves with those we consider better than ourselves; self-esteem is negatively affected. We all have a model in the head, a term of comparison that we have built by looking at years of magazines, advertising, and movies with perfect Hollywood princesses. The mantra must become one and only one: there is no need for me to compare myself to that model because everybody is a unique, generous specimen, rich in the indications of what I am.

Life would be much simpler and happier if we could accept ourselves as we are. A lot of negative emotions would be released, we would have less stress, and more of the things that really matter come into view. The bottom line is, if we really need to change something, we can't do it until we make peace with the current state. This is a vicious circle.

The mind works, in effect, in a strange way. If we resist something, we get more of it.

After all, if we focus our attention on what is bad, we reinforce the bad. And what we pay the most attention to as we think about something will come true.

Everything that comes from you that relates to you is just yours: your feelings, your voice, your actions, your ears, your thighs, your hopes and fears. That's why you are unique. Be happy that you are different from anyone, that you look the way you do and that it is just you. Start to feel that it's your own body, not something separate that you need to live with.

Do you want your house to be just like anyone else's? Or do you love the little things that carry memories? Don't you love the atmosphere of your messy place after playing with your kids? And the plain curtain that you know you should replace, but which your mom sewed and looks so good? Or the piece of furniture that everyone says you should throw out, but you insist on it?

That's how you should feel about your body. You should understand that you don't need to compare it with anyone else's because it's impossible to compare unique things. In addition, who determines what beautiful and ugly mean? You should not compare your body to the celebrities' perfect-looking bodies. First, because they are adjusted with Photoshop and other programs, and they are not real. Second, because you are different, as is everybody.

You're not them. You are neither the next-door girl who, after three children, looks like she did at twenty, nor your friend who you think is gorgeous. You should not only accept your body, but you should fall in love with it. Do you think like Bonnie? Do you think no one could love you because you have some extra weight? Then ask yourself the following questions. Could you fall in love with someone only if they are perfect looking? Would you really love someone because of their body?

Do we really love perfect looking people? I bet you prefer your imperfect companion instead of a perfect looking bodybuilder. You like the little faults of your wife, husband, kids, and friends because they belong to you too. We love imperfections better than perfections.

214

See? We don't measure people based on their weight. In addition, if you are happy with your body and your existence, it will also manifest in your radiance.

How should you love your body?

Here's an exercise that can help those who struggle to be happy about their own imperfections. You have to stand in front of a large mirror and look at yourself as if you were doing it for the first time in your life, like never before, taking time for yourself. It must be a constructive and very careful observation. No distractions, no work commitments, no notification to pull your attention. Only you and the mirror. Next time you hate your body or any part of your body, stand in front of a mirror and look at yourself. Go from top to bottom and sort out your "mistakes". You will have to start looking at yourself from head to toe, objectively observing all the details, without comparisons or judgments.

• Remember what that part of your body has done for you. When did it help, when did it protect you, when did it do something physically useful for you? Say thank you for something that was of help to you. Learn to practice gratitude.

• Appreciate what you have and love your inner self. Don't let a scale or a size define your identity and skills. It is no use to criticize yourself fiercely when looking in the mirror.

Here are some ways to cultivate enormous gratitude in everyday life. When faced with a negative situation, do not be discouraged. Ask yourself instead what you can learn for the future and for reasons to feel grateful. Promise yourself not to be negative or not to criticize yourself for three days. If you make a mistake, forgive yourself and go on your way. This exercise will help you understand that negative thoughts are just a waste of energy. Every day list the reasons why you feel grateful. The body is a miracle and you should celebrate all the gifts it has given you. Think about the goals you have passed, your relationships and the activities you love it was your body that allowed you to do all this. Take note of it every day. Go to the next body part and do the same.

When you have reached your toes, return to your head again, to your face, and now, going downhill, just say to all your body parts, "I love you." Even if you feel a little stupid about it, don't stop. You see, you're going to have a completely different relationship with your appearance. And by the way, let's not forget, it's not a coincidence that it's called outer. What's inside is more important. But what's inside is visible outside. So, use your inner self to love your outer, and you will be much calmer, happier, more satisfied and more confident.

Set the alarm and watch yourself for at least 40 minutes at a time. Doing so could change your life. Experts talk about the epidemic spread of body image disorder; a severe problem that leads us to see ourselves as inadequate every time we look at our body. According to research, 90.2% of women have an altered image of themselves and are not satisfied with their bodies, a fact that has a lot to do with how we look in the mirror. The mirror is your new weapon: from enemy to ally but learning to use it in the right way (Ferrer, 2015).

Compliment yourself. You should consider yourself and treat yourself with the same kindness and the same admiration that you would reserve for those you love. You probably wouldn't direct the same criticisms you do to yourself, to another person. Don't hesitate to compliment yourself, don't be too hard on yourself and forgive yourself when you make a mistake. Get rid of the hatred you feel for yourself, replace it with greater understanding and appreciation. Look in the mirror and repeat: "I am attractive. I am sure of myself. I am fantastic!" Do it regularly and you'll begin to see yourself in a positive light. When you reach a goal, be proud. Look in the mirror and say, "Great job, I'm proud of myself."

Stay away from negativity. Avoid people who only talk badly about their bodies. You risk getting infected by their insecurities and dwelling on your faults. Life is too short and valuable to be consumed by hating yourself or looking for every little fault, especially when the perception you have of yourself tends to be much more critical than that of others. If a person starts to criticize their body, don't get involved in their negativity. Change the subject instead or leave. Wear comfortable clothes that reflect who you are. Everything you have in the wardrobe should enhance your body. Don't wear uncomfortable clothes just to impress others. Remember that those who accept themselves always look great. Wear clean, undamaged garments to dress the body the way you deserve. Buy matching briefs and bras, even though you are the only one to see them. You will remind your inner self that you are doing it exclusively for yourself.

Ask others what they love about you and what they consider your best qualities. This will help you develop yourself and remind you that your body has given you so much. You will probably be surprised to discover what others find beautiful about you; you have probably forgotten about them.

Surround yourself with people who love themselves. People absorb the attitudes and behaviors of the people around them. If your life is full of positive influences, you will also adopt them, and they will help you to love both your inner and outer. Look for optimistic people who work hard to achieve their goals and respect themselves.

Think of all the people who have reached important goals and whom you admire. They can be individuals you know personally or not. They are probably renowned and respected for the goals achieved regardless of the type of physique they have. Take the opportunity to remember that the body is not an obstacle to living or finding happiness. The body can help you pursue all your dreams and desires.

Think of your family, your closest friends, or a person you don't know personally but have always admired. Make a list of their best qualities. Then ask yourself if the image they have of themselves or their bodies has positively influenced their successes or prevented them from reaching a goal.

How to Use Thought Power, Visualization, And Affirmations?

Envision is the mystery

How unmistakably you can envision your proposed result, objective, conviction, propensity, or point of view, decides your degree of enthusiastic connection to your plan. The clearer the vision, the speedier you will have the option to vibrate on a recurrence like anything you desire to accomplish or achieve.

On the off chance that for example you need to accomplish wellbeing bounty, picturing yourself as a solid individual, eating right, working out, being content with your life and seeking after your motivation will immediately change your vibrations in addition to how you feel towards your wellbeing. Since the representation will be certain, your vibrations will be sure and, in this manner,, you are almost certain to draw in better or improved wellbeing.

Similarly, if in the wake of investigating musings comparative with a particular aspect of your life (this should originate from contemplation or journaling), you discover that an idea, for example, "I will never succeed" has no premise in truth and along these lines requires supplanting with a positive idea, for example, "I effectively draw in progress into my life," picturing yourself as fruitful.

The more nitty gritty the representation—what does the riches feel like, how has your life changed, what would you be able to see and hear around you, and so forth.— will demonstrate compelling in view of which, the consequences of the confirmation will be quick. It will initially change the manner in which you consider achievement and afterward change the means you take to make progress in your own and expert life.

Remember that while the inner mind is vastly, it does not have the capacity to separate reality from cause conviction and will to subsequently decipher your representations as your world, the impact of which will be a difference in your vibrational vitality.

Reiteration is the mystery fixing

We have referenced this at different occurrences in the book and will keep doing as such at different territories. For your certifications to impact the change you need, you genuinely need to rehash them whatever number occasions as would be prudent—in any event, when rehashing an attestation causes you to feel like a misrepresentation in view of the distinctions in the orderly situation in your life.

To utilize the intensity of thought viably, couple your insistences with perception and each time your recurrent your attestation, re-run your representation as well and do as such with conviction (confidence) and meticulousness.

Rehashed reliably, your psychological scenes will lead your inner mind and oblivious personalities to have faith in the truth of these scenes so that at long last, your world changes to coordinate your psychological scenes.

Some portion of the purpose behind this impact has to do with the very truth that the inner mind knows no distinction among genuine and envisioned encounters. The other explanation is that redundancy changes your neural pathway. The more you rehash something, the more psyche and oblivious it becomes.

The more you rehash your assertions, perception, activities, circumstances, objectives, wants, propensities, and articles, the more lively they become; the more vivacious they become, the simpler it becomes to show these wants, objectives, propensities, circumstances, and convictions on the material plane (your physical reality).

NOTE: The conviction that attestations don't work regularly breeds from eagerness: you must show restraint. Indication isn't a short-term sensation; it requires time and responsibility. Your desire (in the quest for attesting what you need), truthfulness and confidence in what you are certifying tallies; along these lines, does your regard for the assertion and the time you put into confirming it.

Recall that as we have stated, when you rehash something frequently enough, regardless of whether fortunate or unfortunate, whatever you are rehashing approaches changing the neuronal associations in your brain.

These progressions achieve conviction, conduct, and propensity changes. At the point when these progressions begin occurring, the vitality you vibrate corresponding to a particular aspect of your life improves, and as you currently know, when the vitality in a particular aspect of your life is certain, you draw in inspiration.

Be that as it may, and this is something you ought to consistently remember, the entirety of this beginnings with familiarity with your most basic contemplations corresponding to a particular aspect of your life. Without this mindfulness and the capacity to contemplate your conditions (counting the one you need to show in your life), rehashing insistences will have next to zero impact, which isn't the ideal result.

Health Affirmations

Constantly insert these assertions into your inner mind and your condition of wellbeing will change or improve. Imbedded into the psyche mind more than once, these attestations can assist you with discussing better with your body to recuperate and accomplish in general mental and physical prosperity.

Recall that the feelings joined to the words are as significant as making the idea constant.

"I am solid."

"All aspects of my body is in immaculate wellbeing."

"My brain and body are partners that work with me for my general great."

"Widespread life power courses through me mending and sustaining all aspects of my body, mind, and being."

"My body capacities well."

"The phones in my body cooperate and rapidly to achieve quick mending."

"My body and brain are accomplices that cooperate to cultivate my general prosperity."

"I am a brilliant beam of positive vitality."

"Since I am thought mindful, I control my contemplations. I develop musings of prosperity which is the reason I harvest prosperity in my day by day life."

"My body and brain are my most noteworthy partners. They effectively speak with me about what I have to carry on with an existence of good wellbeing and in general prosperity."

"My wellbeing is my most noteworthy wellspring of riches, which is the reason I love it and take great consideration of it through brain and body sustenance (positive reasoning, food, exercise and nourishment)."

"The associations between my brain and body are away from of correspondence."

"I love my body. I generally give it what it needs to recuperate rapidly and proficiently."

"Through idea mindfulness, I control my wellbeing and prosperity by guaranteeing the considerations generally regular in my brain are solid."

"Great wellbeing is my propensity. I support and care for my body each moment of consistently."

"Consistently all around, I am more beneficial and more grounded."

"I am in flawless wellbeing."

"My body realizes how to fix and recuperate itself."

"My prosperity musings are solid. They blossom into my existence as immaculate wellbeing."

"I am appreciative for flawless wellbeing and generally prosperity as I progress in the direction of satisfying my most noteworthy potential."

Recollect that the feelings you append to the confirmation matters as well. Append feelings of prosperity, joy, great wellbeing, and instinct about your life as you seek after your motivation).

Positive Thinking Affirmations

A positive brain is a reproducing ground for a positive life. Truth be told, to utilize assertions to impact and change any aspect of your life, you first need to turn into a positive scholar. Like most things worth seeking after or having, positive reasoning is a propensity that you can create by immersing your cognizant and subliminal brain with positive words, expressions and sentences/assertions.

The following are 20 inspiration slanted certifications:

"I am an energy magnet."

"Positive musings immerse my psyche."

"I draw in energy."

"I am not my conditions; I make my conditions."

"I am sound, well off, upbeat, and satisfied."

"I have confidence in my capacities and possibilities."

"I am solid willed and versatile."

"I am a champion."

"I spread inspiration wherever I go and to everybody I meet."

"I draw in into my life constructive conditions and individuals."

"I can conquer whatever life tosses at me."

"My brain, body, and soul are vessels for all-inclusive life power."

"My brain, body, and soul feed on positive vitality."

"I and only I control how I feel. I generally decide to feel energy and satisfaction in any event, when life appears to be troublesome."

"I firmly put stock in my capacities. The main individual I contrast myself with is the individual I was yesterday."

"Imaginative energies flood through me each snapshot of the day and carry with them huge amounts of new, inventive thoughts for my life, business, and profession."

"Satisfaction and energy are decisions I decide to encounter each moment of my cognizant existence."

"I have an inherently evolved capacity to defeat negative contemplations, overcome my feelings of dread, and outperform my cutoff points."

"I am an adored offspring of the universe. The universe consistently attempts to guarantee my general prosperity."

"Everything that transpires has a reason. Because of the fact that it transpires, it occurs for me as well."

With regards to positive assertions, make sure to remember that they ought to be only that: positive. This in this way implies as you make certifications for energy (to improve your positive reasoning and cultivate an idealistic attitude), you should introduce arrange your confirmations and ensure the wording is likewise positive.

Affirmations for Improved Self-Image

Poor mental self-view (or self-perception) creates out of a despise for oneself. At its very heart, a poor mental self-portrait is a side effect of self-loathing. Self-loathing is a negative character attribute that you can counter with positive confirmation equipped towards improving your relationship with your body.

The accompanying insistences will help with precisely that. As expressed, and showed prior, you can make mental self-view insistences that mix your feelings and persuade in your present greatness (to trust you are available similarly as you seem to be).

"I am perfectly and brilliantly made."

"I am ideal similarly as I am at this moment."

"I am an appealing individual who draws in constructive individuals and makes ideal conditions throughout my life."

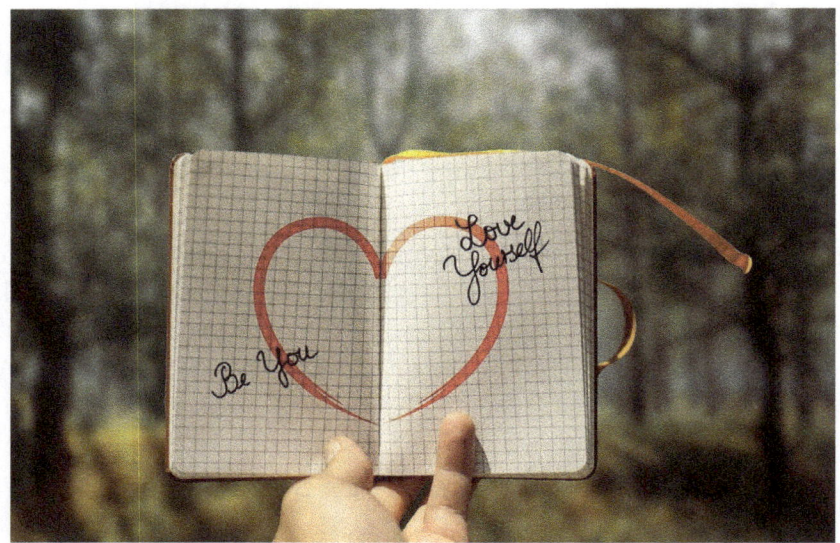

High Self Esteem Hypnosis

Ensure you're in a truly agreeable situation in a spot where you can without much of a stretch tune out the outside world...this meeting merits your complete consideration.

On the off chance that you'd like, you may close your eyes at whenever...

A few people may state that certainty is something that you are simply brought into the world with and on the off chance that you don't have it, you never will...

In any case, this is basically false...

On the off chance that you feel an absence of certainty, you should simply rehearse it during your time ... Much the same as preparing a muscle... these are a few different ways to do this, improving your life drastically.

Take in and inhale out ...

You are sure that you can inhale profoundly at whatever point you wish ... this is a similar conviction that exists in everybody ... It just should be developed and supported to be brought to the surface...

With your imagination, achieve a picture of what the ideal stance of a very sure individual resembles...

How are the shoulders being hung on the group of somebody who is exceptionally certain about themselves?

How does the head balance on the spine of somebody who realizes they can accomplish anything they put commitment towards?

Presently envision yourself holding a similar stance, as though you were taking a gander at an image of yourself or maybe a video...

See your neck stretched supporting the head effortlessly...

Feel the intensity of having your chest open and raised... ready to inhale completely...

Notice how your feet are immovably bound to the ground until you choose to walk, at that point your legs make it easy to move effortlessly along...

At the point when you have certainty, conversing with individuals is pleasant... and others anticipate hearing what's at the forefront of your thoughts...

So, observe yourself now unmistakably conversing with a friend or family member easily... maybe you can envision disclosing to them a smart thought you are having... notice how they react to you with deference and interest to know more...

Presently grow this picture and see yourself talking in a similar way as you were with your companion, yet you are conversing with a little gathering of individuals and they're enthralled by your substance...

Notice how it's ideal to talk for all to hear and communicate what makes you energetic about existence... when you are addressing this gathering of audience members you realize without a doubt that they are getting a charge out of the manner in which you string your words together...

Seeing your stance again before this gathering... shoulders are loose and back... head is held high and your jawline is somewhat raised... an exceptionally delicate grin stays all over as effective words stream out from your mouth as effectively as musings...

Presently observe yourself wrapping up this little assembling and thank others for giving you their full focus... they genuinely express how they are pleased to have seen your certainty and have gained much from all you've needed to state...

We are sure when we acknowledge what our identity is, so at this moment, see your body in the entirety of its excellence, precisely as it was conceived... and acknowledge it...

Your body is your profound vehicle, so you keep up this natural machine by keeping up a sound life.

You feel an increase in certainty each time you disapprove of low quality nourishment, and yes to wellbeing... you feel an ascent in certainty each time you exercise, and propel yourself past the agony and challenge when working out... life feels better on the opposite side of sure decisions...

You feel your certainty fabricating each time you step directly into a dread, instead of fleeing from it... accomplishing something you would prefer not to do in light of the fact that you realize it will improve you is your new super force...

Converse with that individual you've been excessively bashful to previously...

Go after that position you didn't think you were adequate for...

Let's assume you will accomplish more, and make it your need to adhere to your promise...

Go to that get-together despite the fact that you experience social tension every now and then...

You will be glad that you took on something you figured you proved unable... this is the means by which you construct certainty...

Disapprove of that coldblooded desiring that is advising you to eat garbage rather than sustenance...

Move when nobody else is moving... or if nothing else weave your head...

There is a chance to construct trust in any circumstance...

Take a decent full breath in and envision yourself currently, before a huge horde of individuals with an amplifier anticipating your words...

The group is quieted in anticipating your discourse... you see the graciousness that is upon every individual face...

Presently is your chance to be the exemplification of certainty...

Notice your stance, you are holding yourself with respect and poise...

As you convey your message, with a similar dedication you were conversing with your cherished one with, sentences are spilling out of you like a perfectly clear cascade... the words you pick are relentless...

227

you are having an effect on every individual, except considerably more along these lines, in general of humankind...

You are energetic, you are insightful, unadulterated certainty is a characteristic state for you...

[Pause for 30 seconds]

You've said your last, and most impressive words, and a thunder of adulation fills the air...

There is by all accounts a grin evoked on each face you can observer... you can even feel their veritable love for you...

Presently permit this picture to blur, yet hold how it causes you to feel... until the end of time...

Presently hear yourself saying these insistences:

"I am certain"

"I address others effortlessly"

"My stance oozes certainty"

"Others appreciate tuning in to me similarly as I appreciate addressing them"

"Nothing can prevent me from being confident"

"It is simple for me to go to parties and have a ball while I'm there."

"I look for any chance to turn out to be increasingly sure and all the more certain about myself."

"I make a point to hold my head high in any circumstance."

Permit these words to dive deep inside all degrees of your being.

You are sure... you have consistently been... you overlooked... as of recently...

Ascend from your reflection at whatever point you are prepared, and it would be ideal if you practice these strategies day by day and for an amazing duration.

Hypnotherapy for Deep Sleep

Sleep is incredibly important, but sometimes falling asleep can be difficult if we are not in the right mindset.

For this activity, we are going to take you through a visualization that will help ensure that you can get a deep sleep. It's important before falling asleep to relax your mind so that you can travel gently throughout your brain.

Start by noticing your breath. Breathe in through your nose and out through your mouth. This is going to help calm you down so that you can breathe easier.

Begin by breathing in for five and out for five as we count down from twenty. Once we reach one, your mind will be completely clear. Each time a thought passes in, you will think of nothing. You will have nothing in your sight, and you will only think with your mind.

Make sure that you are in a comfortable place where you can sink into the space around you. Let your body become heavy as it falls into the bed. Keep your eyes closed and see nothing in front of you but darkness.

Each time a thought comes in, keep pushing it away. Breathe in through your nose and out through your mouth.

Remember to breathe in for five and out for five. Keep an empty mind and be ready to travel through a journey that will take you to a restful place.

You see nothing in front of you, it is completely dark, and you feel your body lifting gently up like a feather. You are light against the bed, and nothing is keeping you down. Continue to feel your body rise higher and higher. You are floating in space. There's black nothingness around you. You are gently drifting around.

You can see a few stars dotting the sky so far away, but for the most part, you see nothing. You feel yourself slowly moving through space. Your body is light and free, and nothing is keeping you strapped down. You're not afraid in this moment.

You are simply feeling easy and free. Breathe in and out, in and out.

You start to drift more towards a few planets, throughout your journey in space. You can see now that you are up in the highest parts of the galaxy. You see out of the corner of your eye that you can catch a glimpse of Earth. You start gently floating towards it, having to put no effort in at all as your body is like a space rock floating through the stars.

Nothing is holding you down.

Nothing is violently pushing you either. Everything that you feel is a gentle and free emotion. You get closer and closer to Earth now and can see all the clouds that surround you. You start to move down, and you gently enter into the cloud area. Normally gravity would pull you down so fast, but right now you're just simply a gentle body drifting through the air. You get closer and closer to the land. You can see some birds here and there and a few cars and lights on the ground beneath you.

You pass all of this. Gently floating over a sleepy town.

Look down and let your mind explore what it that you see down there is. What is it that is in front of your eyes? What do you notice about this world around you as you continue to go closer and closer to home?

You are gently drifting throughout the sky. You can see trees beneath you. Now, if you reached your hand down, you'd even be able to gently feel a few leaves on the tops of the tallest trees. You don't do this now because you're just concerned with continuing to float through the sky. That's all that you care about in this moment.

You're getting closer and closer and closer to home now, almost ready to fall asleep. You start to see that there is a lake.

You gently float down to the surface of the lake, and you land right in a boat. Your body is a little bit heavier now. You feel it relax into the bottom of the boat. Nothing around you is concerning you right now. You feel no stress or tension in any part of your body. You are simply floating through this space now.

The boat starts to drift on the lake gently. It is dark out now and you look up and see all the stars in the sky. All of this reminds you of the place that you were just a few moments ago. You start to drift closer and closer to sleep.

Do you feel as the tension leaves your body? You are peaceful throughout. You are not holding on to anything that causes you stress or anxiety. You are at ease in this moment. Everything feels good and you have no fear. You drift around in the water now for a little bit longer. You can see everything so clearly in this night sky. Just because it is dark does not mean that it's hard to see. The moon casts a beautiful glow over everything around you. You can feel the moon charging your skin. As you drift closer and closer to sleep, you feel almost nothing in your body now. You continue to focus on your breathing. You are safe, and you are at peace. You are calm, and you are relaxed. You feel incredible in this moment.

The boat starts to lift from the water. You feel as it gets higher above the water. You are even heavier now. Now you are completely glued to this comfortable surface as the boat starts to fly through the sky. You can look down and see that the city beneath you has drifted to sleep. You're getting closer and closer to home now. You can see your home beneath you. The boat gently takes you to your front door, and you float right in. No need to walk or climb stairs. You simply float in and straight to your bed.

You fall delicately into your bed with your head resting nicely on a pillow.

Here you are, in this moment, so peaceful and so relaxed. You are completely at ease. There's nothing that stresses you out or causes any anxiety or tension now. You are simply a body that is trying to fall asleep.

As we count down from 20, you will drift off to sleep. You will be in a very relaxed state where nothing stresses you out. You're not concerned with things that happened in the past, and you aren't going to stay up in fear of what might happen tomorrow, you are asleep. You are relaxed.

Breathe in and out. Breathe in and out.

Meditative Guide for Insomnia

Guided meditation is the form of meditation you engage in with the help of a tutor, or instructor. Ensure that you will not be disturbed, during this meditation.

-       Lay down on your back, preferably on your bed or mat. Make sure you are comfortable on whatever you are lying on.

-       Close your eyes and prepare your mind for the meditation you are about to engage in.

-       Breathe in and out, ensure that your breathing out is audible such that it looks like you are breathing out heavily. Make your body feel the heaviness, after which your body will be relaxed.

-       Pay more attention to your breathing, and you feel easiness. A natural breathing processes.

-       At this point, you will feel your body is relaxed. Feel the way your breath travels through your lungs and hold your breath. As this is happening, you will begin to feel relaxation in your body.

-       You can begin to breathe normally right now, and as you breathe you feel your muscles, joints, and back relaxed.

-       Pay more attention to your stomach area right now, where your abdominal muscles are present. Tighten the muscles in your abdomen and hold your breath for 10 seconds and release your muscles. During this release, feel the difference the tightness of your abdominal muscle and the relaxation of these muscles.

-       Repeat the above process 5 times.

-       Breathe in and out, tighten your abdomen and release it to relaxation.

Feet

- Divert your attention to your feet and make them relaxed. The relaxation should be from your toes to your ankles. Tighten your toes and feet and feel them become heavy and relaxed.

- Focus on your nails, feel them relaxed and let go.

- Pay attention to your thigh area and feel them relaxed.

- Again, focus on your waist, lower and upper back, joints and feel them relaxed. You will feel the feel heavy, and very relaxed

Upper limbs

- At this point, focus your attention on your arms. Feel them heavy and relaxed.

- Get a sense of how heavy your arm is, and feel the relaxation shift to your elbow, wrist, and fingers become very relaxed.

Face, neck and facial muscles

- Shift your focus to your facial muscles, neck and face.

- Every muscle in your face, your cheeks and chin become relaxed, and your entire body is now relaxed.

A deeper meditation for the abdomen

- Locate your center, which is your abdominal region. Imagine there is a bowl on your abdomen. Slowly see the bowl rolling over your abdomen area, and it relaxes every muscle the bowl rolls in contact with.

- The bowl now moves slowly from your abdomen area to your right hip carefully and softly massaging the muscles of the hips it comes in contact to.

- Massaging back and forth all the muscles in your abdomen.

- The ball continues to roll over to your knee, and around your knee. You can feel the tension on your navel melting away. Roll the ball slowly to your toe, and over to your toes, from your small toes to the big toes.

Every part of your body this ball comes in contact with feel the part of your body relaxing.

- Now feel the ball begins to roll upwards away from your toes again. Massaging and reducing tension around your toes, knees, ankles and rolls over to your center, your abdominal area.

- Again, this balls rolls to your left thigh, and your knee, massaging both the back and front of your knee.

With your ball you move this ball to wherever you choose, and how long you want it to be.

- With this ball, massage your knee, and ankle and toes. This ball touches every muscle in your toes, it gently massages them and at this point, you feel your muscle relax.

- Feel the ball roll back up your leg, your knee and thigh muscle and arriving back at your center.

- Shift the focus of the ball to the base of your spinal cord. Allow the ball rest there for 5 seconds, and allow it to move up your spine, and near your heart. At this point, you can feel the ball massaging the internal organs in your body. The ball massages the heart, and you feel relaxed.

- The ball rolls to your throat area, and the back of your neck area. You feel your neck area relaxing after the ball massages it. You feel tension reducing around your neck area.

- The ball travels down your arm, and to your wrist. The ball gently massages your wrist, and fingers.

- You feel the ball roll up your arm, to your shoulder and neck. It travels down to your elbow, forearm, and wrist and into the palm of your hands.

- Allow the ball gently to massage your palm, and fingers. The ball moves up your arm, shoulder and face and as it reaches up in your face, the ball splits into a hundred tiny balls. You feel them travel around your face, to your eyes, eyebrow, cheeks, chin, teeth, tongue and teeth.

- You feel the ball massaging your face and every part of your face. At this point, you should enjoy this facial massage.

- I want you to imagine as you are lying down the ceiling of your house. Your eyes are still closed, so imagine the ceiling of your room opening itself up, and the roof also opens itself open.

- Still looking at this opening, you will see the beautiful white sky. The sky is clear, bright, and the moon is out and also full, filled with stars. This is a magical peaceful night. You are alone, safe in the beautiful part of your house.

- Watch the twinkling and beautiful little stars, looking down on you and you are enjoying the peace of the night.

- You look again at the stars, the little ones that are thousands of miles away are not shining so beautiful like the big star closer to you that is looking at you directly from the sky.

- You are looking deep into galaxy, beyond time, you see a million other stars waiting for you and shining at you.

- Take a deep breath. breathe in a rich air from the infinite and beautiful galaxy filled with stars.

- Feel yourself been a part of these stars, there is no separation between you and them. Feel you are already a part of this wonderful galaxy.

- As you experience this, you become a shooting star, shining across the galaxy like others.

- Slowly you begin to fade into the sky, into the everlasting space and galaxy.

- You are living in the wonders of this space, where there is neither time, past or future. You feel you are the stars, the moon, and you occupy the pace between the planets.

- You are floating off slowly, as you travel across this universe; you feel your body wants to drift away. You feel peace, wholeness, and love.

- When you are ready, and feel relaxed, you can let go of the galaxy. When you drift off, you will drift into a peaceful and wonderful sleep.

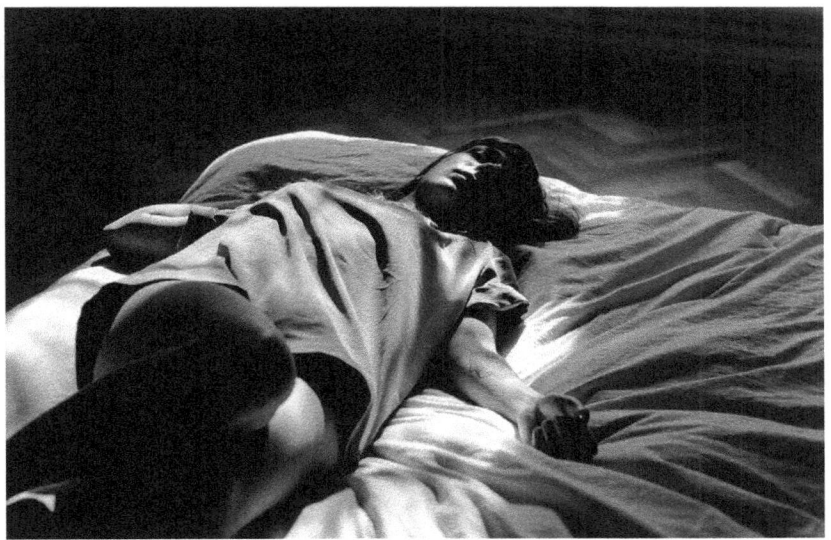

Mindfulness Meditation to Fall Asleep

You are laying in a completely comfortable position right now. Your body is well-rested, and you are prepared to drift deeply into sleep. The deeper you sleep, the healthier you feel when you wake up.

Your eyes are closed, and the only thing that you are responsible for now is falling asleep. There isn't anything you should be worried about other than becoming well-rested. You are going to be able to do this through this guided meditation into another world.

It will be the transition between your waking life and a place where you are going to fall into a deep and heavy sleep. You are becoming more and more relaxed, ready to fall into a trance-like state where you can drift into healthy sleep.

Start by counting down slowly. Use your breathing in fives to help you become more and more asleep.

Breathe in for ten, nine, eight, seven, six, and out for five, four, three, two, and one. Repeat this once more. Breathe in for ten, nine, eight, seven, six, and out for five, four, three, two, and one.

You are now more and more relaxed, more and more prepared for a night of deep and heavy sleep. You are drifting away, faster and faster, deeper and deeper, closer and closer to a heavy sleep. You see nothing as you let your mind wander.

You are not fantasizing about anything. You are not worried about what has happened today, or even farther back in your past. You are not afraid of what might be there going forward. You are not fearful of anything in the future that is causing you panic.

You are highly aware of this moment that everything will be OK. Nothing matters but your breathing and your relaxation. Everything in front of you is peaceful. You are filled with serenity and you exude calmness. You only think about what is happening in the present moment where you are becoming more and more at peace.

Your mind is blank. You see nothing but black. You are fading faster and faster, deeper and deeper, further and further. You are getting close to being completely relaxed, but right now, you are OK with sitting here peacefully.

You aren't rushing to sleep because you need to wind down before bed. You don't want to go to bed with anxious thoughts and have nightmares all night about the things that you are fearing. The only thing that you are concerning yourself with at this moment is getting friendly and relaxed before it's time to start to sleep.

You see nothing in front of you other than a small white light. That light becomes a bit bigger and bigger. As it grows, you start to see that you are inside a vehicle. You are laying on your bed, everything around you are still there. Only, when you look up, you see that there is a large open window, with several computers and wheels out in front of you.

You realize that you are in a spaceship floating peacefully through the sky. It is on autopilot, and there is nothing that you have to worry about as you are floating up in this spaceship. You look out above you and see that the night sky is more gorgeous than you ever could have imagined.

All that surrounds you is nothing but beauty. Bright stars are twinkling against a black backdrop. You can make out some of the planets. They are all different than you would ever have imagined. Some are bright purple, others are blue. There are detailed swirls and stripes that you didn't know were there.

You relax and feel yourself floating up in this space. When you are here, everything seems so small. You still have problems back home on Earth, but they are so distant that they are almost not real. Some issues make you feel as though the world is ending, but you see now that the entire universe is still doing fine, no matter what might be happening in your life. You are not concerned with any issues right now.

You are soaking up all that is around you. You are so far separated from Earth, and it's crazy to think about just how much space is out there for you to explore. You are relaxed, looking around. There are shooting stars all in the distance. There are floating rocks passing by your ship. You are floating around, feeling dreamier and dreamier.

You are passing over Earth again, getting close to going back home. You are going to be sent right back into your room, falling more heavily with each breath you take back into sleep. You are getting closer and closer to drifting away.

You pass over the earth and look down to see all of the beauty that exists. The green and blue swirl together, white clouds above that make such an interesting pattern. Everything below looks like a painting. It does not look real.

You get closer and closer, floating so delicately in your small spaceship. The ride is not bumpy. It is not bothering you.

You are floating over the city now. You see random lights flicker on. It doesn't look like a map anymore like when you are so high above.

You are looking down and seeing that gentle lights still flash here and there, but for the most part, the city is winding down. Everyone is drifting faster and faster to sleep. You are getting closer and closer to your home.

You see that everything is peaceful below you. The sun will rise again, and tomorrow will start. For now, the only thing that you can do is prepare and rest for what might be to come.

You are more and more relaxed now, drifting further and further into sleep.

You are still focused on your breathing; it is becoming slower and slower. You are close to drifting away to sleep now.

When we reach one, you will drift off deep into sleep.

Detox your Emotional State of Mind

With regards to detoxing, you can discover hundreds, if not a large number of sites, books, and articles laying out incalculable approaches to kill contaminations and rinse the body. decent physical detox can be useful whenever done securely, In the same way as other present-day human services experts, brain and body are profoundly associated, so your perspective can profoundly affect your heart and in general wellbeing. In this manner, enthusiastic detoxing is similarly as significant as physical detoxing for ideal wellbeing.

Upsetting feelings like resentment, tension, and wretchedness cause us to feel awful, yet what isn't so evident is the harm that these feelings can have on our physical bodies. The earth-shattering INTERHEART study uncovered that psychosocial factors like pressure and sorrow are similar to hypertension and stomach heftiness with regards to hazard factors for coronary illness. Another investigation drove by Karina W. Davidson, Ph.D., of Columbia University Medical Center shows that upbeat individuals are 22 percent more averse to create coronary illness than their troubled partners.

Although researchers are not so much sure what the immediate connection between negative feelings and heart wellbeing is, inquire about proposes that downturn may expand irritation and cause the blood to cluster all the more rapidly, which can harm veins and thicken supply route dividers. What's more, specialists have since quite a while ago realized that the pressure hormones cortisol and adrenaline increment circulatory strain, pulse, and blood sugars. These consequences for the body can prompt a coronary failure or stroke.

This may appear awful news, particularly thinking that we as a whole vibe angry or upset now and then. In any case, fortunately, we can entirely diminish the measure of negative feelings that we feel on an everyday premise and hence decline the danger of creating cardiovascular issues. Next are a few hints on the most proficient method to do a passionate detox to purge the psyche and the heart.

Know about Your Emotions. The more significant part of us has a characteristic propensity to attempt to abstain from feeling terrible, so we silence our feelings instead of managing them head-on. We may do this by imagining everything is okay when it isn't, denying that a difficulty exists, or going to liquor, food, or T.V. for the interruption. Lamentably, issues, and negative emotions don't only leave. They decay under the surface and will come out sooner or later, not far off. The best activity when you are feeling furious or down is to know about the feelings inside you and permit yourself to contact them altogether.

Get to the Root of Your Feelings. When you have perceived that you are feeling a specific way, the following activity is a wonder why you are feeling that particular feeling. Indeed, it is difficult to accuse others or circumstances of making you upset; in the end, you are the one showing the inclination. As a general rule, negative emotions can be followed back to dread, blame, or outrage with yourself. Attempt to pinpoint the specific reason for your negative sentiments, and from that point, you can detail activity to intend to release those emotions.

Diving profound into your feelings is no simple errand, and you may wind up groping depleted or missing the mark with regards to getting to the foundation of your emotions. An expert specialist can assist you in managing your feelings in a sheltered and effective way, which will leave you with more opportunity to concentrate on the great. Furthermore, dear companions, relatives, and friends and family can be priceless help during a passionate detox.

Implement Powerful Breathing Techniques

Diaphragmatic breathing, or profound breathing from the stomach as opposed to the chest, is an approach to unwind and lessen nervousness of different sorts. Although we are on the whole equipped for breathing along these lines, not many of us do as such in our regular day to day existence.

Significance of Deep Breathing

Profound breathing encourages you to maintain a strategic distance from the "battle or flight" reaction to unpleasant circumstances. In these circumstances, your body's programmed frameworks are on high caution and sign your heart to pulsate quicker and breathing rate to increment. By deliberately getting mindful of your breathing and managing its profundity and speed, the probability of spiraling into a frenzy or nervousness assault is brought down.

The most effective method to Practice Diaphragmatic Breathing

Note: If you live with an ailment, talk with your primary care physician preceding starting any sort of unwinding preparing exercise. It's ideal for rehearsing this breathing example while you are in an unlatched and safe condition at home. Along these lines, you will be bound to utilize this method when confronted with circumstances that trigger side effects of social uneasiness issue (SAD) or different problems with nervousness. The following are the means to take to rehearse profound relaxing:

- Locate a calm spot liberated from interruptions. Lie on the floor or in a seat, relax any tight dress and expel glasses. Rest your hands in a lap or on the arms of the place.

- Breathe in, taking a full breath from your mid-region as you check to three. As you inhale, you will feel your stomach ascend. The hand on your chest ought not to move.

- After a brief delay, gradually breathe out while tallying to three. If you wish, you can say an expression as you breathe out, for example, "quiet."

- Proceed with this example of cadence relaxing for five to ten minutes until you feel loose.

Notwithstanding adhering to these guidelines, consider tuning in to a voice recording, for example, the free MP3 sound document offered by McMaster University, which remembers headings for rehearsing diaphragmatic relaxing. Utilization of a sound account permits you to completely unwind and focus on the method without adhering to composed directions.

Barriers to Practicing Deep Breathing

If you find that you come back to shallow breathing regardless of rehearsing profound breathing, it is the case that you need more practice in various circumstances. Have a go at taking a yoga class that empowers intense breathing or pursue a care contemplation course. Utilizing different methodologies that fuse profound breathing will give you more opportunities to practice and start to ace the craft of breathing from your stomach.

Artists and Deep Breathing

Artists are educated to inhale profoundly while singing to improve the sound of their voice and to maintain a melody without breaking in the center. If you are an artist or artist who plays a breeze instrument and lives with social nervousness, you may profit by rehearsing profound relaxing. Breathing profoundly from your mid-region while performing will assist with forestalling hyperventilation or the inclination that you can't get your breath. If intense breathing alone doesn't appear to improve your tension, consider finding out about and rehearsing these different procedures. You may even locate an on the web or nearby specialist who can direct you through these kinds of activities. For a supportive mentor in your pocket, there is likewise "Woebot," a visit application that can manage you through unwinding practices just as assist you with testing negative idea designs.

A Quick Five-Minute Breathing Exercise

- Set your telephone to go off once every day at a convenient time.

- At the point when the caution goes off, practice profound relaxation for five minutes.

- After the five minutes are up, check whether you feel progressively loose and less on edge.

- After some time, it should turn out to be progressively typical to inhale along these lines steadily.

Breathing profoundly from your stomach is an educated ability. Although, as infants, we as a whole do this intuitively, when you live with tension, it can feel hard to inhale along these lines in a snapshot of frenzy. If, in the wake of rehearsing profound breathing, you, despite everything, feel severe nervousness, consider counseling a psychological wellness expert or clinical specialist for evaluation and proposals for treatment.

Weight Loss Affirmations

Weight loss affirmations are a great way to stimulate your journey to weight loss.

We all know that weight loss is not easy. The use of these weight loss affirmations can help people facing stubborn internal resistance when trying to lose weight.

These are the affirmations that you can suggest yourself while practicing self-hypnosis, cognitive-behavioral theory, or Sleep learning system. In the first two methods, these affirmations can directly be suggested, and in the third method, you can record these and listen to them while sleeping.

You must be careful while choosing theses affirmations. It is suggested that you should select the affirmations that you believe yourself and do not raise an objection when they are suggested to you. The failure happens because if you do not believe yourself, then it will not work for you. Moreover, it is suggested that you use a few affirmations that you think are effective for you. Do not try to suggest all at once. It may retard the effectiveness of the methods. There are also chances that the brain may become confused in case of any two opposite affirmations. So, better select your affirmations very carefully.

Now we will list the affirmations for excessive weight loss:

• Weight loss makes sense to me.

• I want to reach the goal of weight loss.

• I lose weight every day.

• I love to exercise regularly.

• I eat foods that contribute to my health and well-being.

• I only eat when I am hungry.

• I can see myself clearly with my ideal weight.

- I love the taste of healthy food.

- I can control how much I want to eat.

- I like training. I feel better.

- Through exercise, I will be stronger and stronger every day.

- I can reach the ideal weight and maintain it.

- I love and care for my body.

- I deserve a slim, healthy, and attractive body.

- I always have a healthier eating habit.

- I lose weight every day.

- It looks good and feels good.

- I can do what it takes to be healthy.

- I am happy to redefine success.

- I decided to train.

- I want to eat food that looks and feels good.

- I am responsible for my health.

- I love my body.

- I put up with building a better body for myself.

- When I wake up, I have a great time doing exercise every morning to achieve my desired weight loss.

- I am working on a weight loss program by changing my diet from unhealthy to healthy.

- I am happy with everything I do to lose weight.

- I get thinner and healthier every day.

- I am developing an attractive body.

• I develop a lifestyle with life health.

• I can create a body that I will like and enjoy.

These were general affirmations that you can use in a reasonable condition. You can move to more specific affirmations later, when you feel that now it is time to modify my practice. Some of these affirmations are given below that will help you cope up with weight gain with a more specific approach.

• Discovering my unique diet and exercise system for weight loss is exciting.

• I am a beautiful person.

• I am a weight loss success story.

• I am happy to lose 20 pounds.

• I am ready to develop new ideas about myself and my body.

• I choose to trust the ability to make positive changes in my life.

• I congratulate myself on choosing the right food.

• I drink eight glasses of water daily.

• I eat fruits and vegetables every day, mainly chicken and fish.

• I enjoy walking 3-4 times a week and have at least three toning exercised a week.

• I free the need to criticize my body.

• I have a substantial weight in the world due to my low weight.

• I learn and use mental, emotional, and spiritual skills for success. Ready to change!

• I love and appreciate my body.

• I will take care of my body in optimal health.

• I'm happy that I have the ideal weight.

- It feels good to move your body. The practice is fun!

- It's easy to follow a healthy diet plan.

- My lifestyle changes my body.

- My metabolism is excellent.

- My stomach is flat.

- Take a deep breath to relax and deal with stress.

- My efforts are worth reaching the ideal weight.

You can make your own affirmation to that suit your routine and efforts.

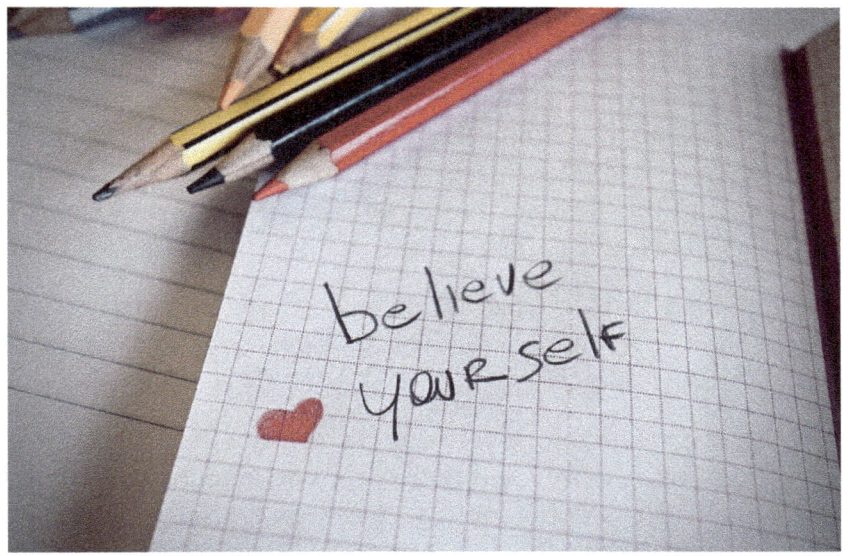

Meaning of Mindfulness

When you come to understand what mindfulness meditation truly means, you will feel a more profound sense of belonging to it. In other words, your perception of it will transcend its surface-value, which is the functional role of helping you to unwind and melt away the stress. Therefore, by getting to know its deeper values, you will find that it is not just an option; it also has an integral part of your daily life.

The generally accepted definition of mindfulness is that it is a mental and emotional process. Specifically, it is the practice of focusing one's thoughts and feelings towards what is happening during the present moment. It is also widely believed that, through the practice of mindfulness meditation, one's ability to focus on the present moment can be strengthened.

Buddhist Beginnings

In Buddhism, the concept of our modern-day understanding of "mindfulness" came from the ancient Pali word "sati," a term that means "to bear in mind" or "to remember" (Pali is an ancient Prakrit language that is used as the liturgical and scriptural language of Theravada Buddhism). Traditionally, sati means to bear in mind and recall the dharma, or the teachings of the Buddha.

Ancient Buddhism further explains that you can understand the process of focusing on the present moment by learning the skandhas, otherwise known as the Five Aggregates.

The Five Aggregates organize your mind's ability of consciousness as influenced by your own pre-conditioned attitudes and past experiences. They are namely the material form, feelings, perceptions, and volition, sensory consciousness.

The Material Form is your physical body and the material elements that surround you, as well as enter and leave your body (such as the air you breathe).

Feelings are the emotional sensations that may be described as pleasant, neutral, or unpleasant.

Perceptions are your sensory awareness of the dimensions of an object, such as the color, shape, size and smell.

Volition refers to the mental, physical and verbal behavior you choose to conduct.

Sensory consciousness is your awareness of the thoughts that occur in your mind and the stimuli that your five senses can take in.

Buddhists explain that these Five Aggregates come in waves as one practice mindfulness meditation. However, you must avoid "clinging" to any of these five aggregates, so you can free yourself from suffering and unleash your true self.

Psychology

In Psychology, mindfulness may be regarded as a practice that can develop the mind's metacognitive abilities. Psychological researchers Kirk Warren Brown, Richard M. Ryan, and J. David Creswell explained that how a person defines mindfulness depends on who that person is and how mindfulness is applied.

According to them, some regard mindfulness as a mental state, while others describe it as a set of skills and strategies. Thus, there should be a clear line between the trait and the state of mindfulness.

Another psychologist, Scott R. Bishop proposed that mindfulness can be defined as a type of "non-elaborative, non-judgmental, present-centered awareness" wherein every thought, sensation and feeling that comes up to one's conscious attention is "acknowledged and accepted as it is."

Brown, however, explained that mindfulness is a quality of consciousness that manifests in – but is not necessarily the same as – the activities through which it is enhanced (such as meditation).

Steven F. Hick, the author of Mindfulness and the Therapeutic Relationship, explained that there are both formal and informal practices of mindfulness. The formal practice is mindfulness meditation, which involves the process of focusing one's attention on sensations, breathing, the body, or anything that takes place in the present moment. The informal practice of mindfulness is when you apply mindfulness in everyday exercises, such as being mindful while doing the dishes, eating, or listening to music.

He further explains that the present is the only moment we ever really have "to be alive in," yet our attention to it is usually neither vivid nor stable. However, by training the mind to pay attention through mindful meditation, we can strengthen our ability to sustain our attention moment by moment.

How Mindfulness Meditation Came to Be

Following is a brief overview on the historical development of mindfulness meditation. By learning about its roots, you can appreciate the practice even more and this will hopefully inspire you to incorporate it into your everyday life.

Mindfulness meditation, as it is today, is founded on the vipassana meditation of Buddhism. The term vipassana means, "to become aware of the present moment as it really is." The practice of vipassana is meant to help one see the true nature of reality, which is the impermanence of things. By becoming aware of impermanence, one can break free or be liberated from desire, which is the actual cause of suffering.

In fact, mindfulness is so important that it is actually the seventh step in the Noble Eightfold Path of Buddhism. To have the right mindfulness is to be conscious of what one is doing in the present moment and never be absent-minded. It is to be aware of the impermanent state of one's body, mind and feelings.

The person who is most responsible for spreading vipassana meditation throughout modern Asia and the West is the Burmese Theravada Buddhist Monk Mahasi Sayadaw U Sobhana (1904 – 1982). His publications and teachings became so widespread that they enabled him to help train over 700,000 meditators. His publications, along with accessibility to the Buddhist sutras, were translated into English, causing the concept of mindfulness meditation to become even more widespread.

A significant proponent of mindfulness meditation in the west is Kabat-Zinn who is a Professor of Medicine Emeritus and was a student of several Buddhist teachers such as Seung Sahn and Thich Nhat Hanh. What made his teaching of mindfulness appealing to the west is his ability to synergize it with science. As a result, his stress reduction program was widely accepted in hospitals and other medical centers.

The movement that Jon Kabat-Zinn started quickly picked up pace and led to the Mindfulness Movement, which has led over 20,000 chronically ill patients as well as a significant number of individuals in peak health to practice mindfulness meditation and allowing them to enhance their quality of life. Thus, mindfulness became a well-known mainstream concept and practice.

Meditation and Mindfulness

Surely many have already heard of mindfulness. A Buddhist relaxation technique that allows us to manage emotions, attitudes, and thoughts better. Thanks to the development of this capacity, we manage life's complicated situations better, without judging ourselves and accepting them as something necessary and from which to learn.

The mindfulness is based on meditation and mindfulness. That is, in a state of absolute relaxation, but conscious, in which we are able to observe ourselves in the present moment. Mindfulness aims to unite our innermost self with the outside world.

The goal is to learn to isolate our feelings from problems. Awareness states that the issues are not life's bad circumstances, but the negative emotions which relate these facts. It's not about suppressing these feelings but learning how to properly manage them so that they don't cause stress and anxiety.

Why practice mindfulness?

You may ask yourself, and why do I need to focus on the present? Why accept the conditions today? Let's understand the significance below.

• Higher Productivity

The contribution to personal efficiency is definitely the undisputed consideration of further examination of present conditions. We are often beset by professional and personal problems, so we can't see potentialities in the scenario.

If we engage in knowledge the mind understands better every aspect of our lives without projecting too far into the future or the past. It is therefore the best technique for those who want to begin to behave productively.

• Improvement of cognitive skills

There are a number of aspects of cognitive skills. The big picture is made up of concentration, memory, comprehension and even social skills. The strategy increases the overall scenario.

If we focus solely on the moment, we tend to only look at what is happening now. The brain is doing the same thing, as a result. You are still learning to understand the sensations of the world in greater detail, which may be crucial to your progress.

- Fighting anxiety and stress

Anxiety and stress are just a few of the evil characteristics that come from our everyday life's hurry and demands. For example, a lot of people use mindfulness to battle harsh working conditions.

In any case, it's interesting to note that the technique also teaches body and mind patience and discipline in addition to providing total focus at the moment. As a consequence, the irritability levels decrease with increasing self-control.

- Self-consciousness and self-improvement

Have you ever stopped paying attention to what you think, your convictions, principles and abilities? The reaction to that is negative for many people. Developing the ability to be conscious is important in such situations.

Awareness practice helps manage internal issues that we don't pay much attention to, summing up the effect.

Simple Ways to Practice Mindfulness in Your Daily Life

Practicing mindfulness is a step towards a better quality of life. However, it is not always easy, because we need to adopt this philosophy of ancestral roots to modern times. To achieve this, we can use several paths and strategies: we need to find the one that best suits our needs, our daily lives.

Admittedly, most of us are drawn to mindfulness, not because it's trendy, not because we've been told about its methods, or because we find it in nearly every book, magazine or self-help article that we read. We are fascinated and enticed because it allows us to see our mind as a mirror from which we can understand the world more deeply, more closely and more clearly. It is innovative, and useful above all.

But, with its responsibilities, its strict routines and our ever-busy look, our daily life drags us along. We can't use a couple of hours a day to learn to meditate, we can't find some free time, and we're telling ourselves that meditation isn't for us.

That's one error. We are closer than ever to mindfulness, and in many different ways. There are those who start at home following a book's instructions or even a course over the internet.

There are also people who can't keep quiet, can't integrate with more people in the dynamics of a community. To them, there's the right to meditate while walking while doing sports.

Mindfulness in modern times, in times of movement

Times change, but not only remain the origins of our culture, our faith, and this extraordinary legacy brought about by mindfulness, but are more important than ever. So, despite our troubled lives ' current uncertainty... When and how can we learn to develop a full consciousness? How do I learn to meditate, relax and touch the here and now?

• Rohan Gunatillake is an author who revolutionizes the field of consciousness with a very specific aspect: creatively and consciously conceiving meditation, thanks to new technology or even sports.

• He discusses how we evolve and how we adjust. Today our needs are more urgent, our worlds turbulent, but our sources of learning are broader: the internet and new technologies bring us closer to the area of personal growth than ever before and also lead us into the realm of meditation.

• Rohan Gunatillake calls this new behavior "social meditation," because the urban environment and our digital society and work culture are what defines us today, even if it scares us. How to take part in a 10-

day retreat and learn to meditate? If not, we've got our own house, work and those wonderful technologies that can teach us how to communicate quickly with our life...

We are all part of the movement, in this dynamic world. We should not be mistaken, however, because perception is also a complex practice: we have become magnificent receivers of the present moment, of each of its wonderful complexities, oscillations, shifts, smells, tastes, sensations....

Some ways to learn mindfulness

Daniel Goleman said focus is a muscle that we have to work on a daily basis to be more open to what surrounds us and what is happening within us. But... how can we do it if we have hardly enough time? Can we really learn to meditate once a week, by taking a class?

Many people will certainly do it, but many of them go out of curiosity to these classes and end up giving up after a few days because it doesn't work, because they can't control their fickle mind and find the perfect balance in the context where everything else is in.

Nevertheless, if this custom of Buddhist origin came to the West more than 2,500 years old, it was no mistake. Many scientists like Dr. Kabat-Zin and many others have realized that our stressful world is speeding us up, and so we need the support and benefits of being conscious. We have numerous options, shapes and pathways to start this exercise.

Mindfulness at Work

Organizations such as Apple, Google, Adidas or eBay are already taking their daily lives into account. For this technique to be successful, of course, we definitely need an atmosphere and a labor policy that encourages its adoption, but in fact it's not that complicated to achieve. Those guidelines would be:

• Start working without urgency (you may not be able to do it in the first week, but it will be possible to do it little by little)

- Take 5 minutes to settle down, plan the day; remember what you need to do and how you feel.

- Breathe deeply and become aware of your body, postures and potential stresses, here and now.

- Take a 5-minute break to meditate every 40 minutes, to relax, and to reconnect.

Meditate while walking

Ideally, we can walk every day for half an hour of sun, walk at a fast pace for half an hour and wear comfortable clothing. The aim is not only to train our body but also our mind on the basic principles of being mindful. The key criteria would be these:

- Start to walk at normal pace. You will slowly find the rhythm that is most soothing, cathartic and freeing for you. There are people who prefer a slow pace and others who want to get going more quickly.

- At some point it's time to focus your attention. Visualize your mind as a spotlight that guides your light at one particular point and then another: first at your breath, then at the sensation of your feet as they touch the ground, the breeze caressing your skin... Focus your attention on those points. Cyclically: first, and then, second.

- You will notice, little by little, that you no longer need to focus your attention on your body at each of these points. After a few days, your flashlight's concentration will be so broad that you will notice everything at once.

The Mindfulness at Home

- Choose a space, place, and time of day that best suits your needs for meditation. Remember that you must commit firmly and willingly because it must be continuous work.

- Start with 10 or 15 minutes. Gradually, as you adjust, you can meditate longer.

- Choose the technique that best suits your needs.

- Be patient and don't expect immediate results. Mindfulness requires time and commitment.

Times change and we will always have such an exciting and valuable activity within reach, given our complex and challenging lives. We just need to find the path which fits best, which is most convenient and close to us. Let's expand our perspectives and take a step towards understanding what consciousness is bringing us.

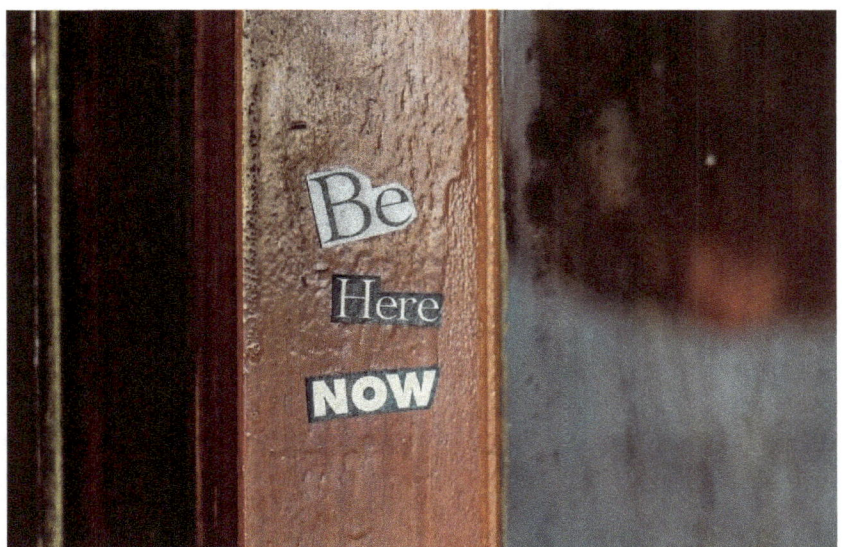

Different Forms of Mindfulness

It is interesting to note, as we delve deeper into the concept of mindfulness, that although the birth of the idea is pegged as being from Buddhist practices, this is predominantly because Buddhist practices are some of the most ancient. While mindfulness is in no way a religious practice, it is a spiritual practice and it is one that exists in many forms in many different organized religions and spiritual followings.

For example, prayer, which is common to almost all organized religions, is a form of mindfulness. By understanding this, you may find it easier to accept that mindfulness is not simply some hyped-up New Age practice. It is an ancient way to communicate with our higher selves. It is also important to note that although we will discuss meditation and yoga as techniques which can help to improve mindfulness, these should not be considered barriers to practicing mindfulness if these activities are not available to you for any reason.

It is vital that we understand that anyone, in any circumstances, with any capacity and in any society can practice mindfulness. Although we are talking about it more now, there are entire groups of people who have always practiced mindfulness simply as part of their everyday lives because this what was handed down through their generations. This does not, therefore, preclude anyone who may have grown up in a different setting or culture to practicing mindfulness. This is not an "us" and "them" practice, it is a "we," as the human race, practice (What is mindfulness, 2015).

There are five forms of mindfulness techniques which can be practiced in isolation or, when the techniques become easier for you to manage, simultaneously. The five techniques we will discuss here are: basic mindfulness meditation, body sensation mindfulness, sensory mindfulness, emotional mindfulness and urge surfing (Different Types of Mindfulness, n.d.)

Basic Mindfulness Meditation

For the sake of explanation, a basic mindfulness meditation consists of sitting quietly while focusing on your breathing or repeating a mantra you find helpful for focus.

While in this state, you will acknowledge thoughts without judgement and allow them to pass through you so that you can return to your breathing or mantra. There are no rules about where and when this can be practiced. In general, you want to select a place that has few sensory distractions. It is also best to ensure that your body is using as little energy as possible at the time, so by sitting or laying down, you can conserve your body's energy and use it to practice your focus.

Body Sensation Mindfulness

Mentally scan your body from head to toe, acknowledging any twitch, pain or twinge in that body part and then move on to the next, working your way up your entire body. Some areas may need more time than others.

If you know that you suffer from an ailment in a specific part of your body, you can spend more time focusing on that part but be aware of doing so with a negative connotation. This exercise is to practice shifting your focus while staying committed to the task at hand.

Sensory Mindfulness

In this mindfulness technique, you will acknowledge the information you are receiving from your senses, label it as the sense from which it comes and move on from it. For instance, the voice of an angry customer over the phone should not be labelled with the emotions you believe it represents or the possible consequences of their complaint, but it should be labelled simply as sound, acknowledged and allowed to move on. The bright lights of an oncoming vehicle at night is not selfishness on the part of the other driver or dangerous if you become momentarily blinded to the road ahead, the headlights are simply labelled as light and allowed to move on.

You can also sit quietly and try to switch between senses, focusing only on the information you are receiving through that sense. You may be amazed at how many sounds and sights you miss when you are attempting to take everything in at once.

Emotional Mindfulness

In this mindfulness technique we acknowledge emotions as they enter our minds and name them for what they are without judgement. By not judging emotions, we are not labelling them as positive or negative, the emotion is present, acknowledged, named and allowed to move on. If it makes it easier for you, you can greet the emotion with words. For instance, "Hello irritation. I see and acknowledge you," and then, "Goodbye irritation. You are not relevant to this moment."

Urge Surfing

This technique is useful in dealing with addictions or compulsive urges. Instead of waiting for the craving to go away, acknowledge the craving and be aware of how it feels when the craving is in your body. Use your curiosity and the other techniques mentioned here to label and acknowledge without judgement any emotion or body sensation which may arise in connection to this craving and then allow the craving to move on. The most important key to urge surfing is, as the name suggests, ride the wave of the urge without allowing it to engulf you. Awareness is vital here.

It may be tempting to try and replace the urge with something else or distract yourself. This is not helpful in the long run though, as those distractions may not always be available to you.

Sharing the Idea

This is not a mindfulness technique but a step which may result from practicing and enjoying mindfulness. When you are enjoying the benefits of mindfulness you will most likely want to share this practice with others. This is a wonderful idea but needs to be approached from the correct mindset. Just as mindfulness asks us not to judge the thoughts and emotions that enter our minds, we should be careful not to judge other forms or techniques of mindfulness practice, with which we may not be familiar. We would be remiss to assume that because someone else is practicing prayer instead of meditation in the form you know it, that they are somehow not still practicing mindfulness. If someone becomes mindful through hiking or jogging rather than yoga, that is their journey, it may not be yours, but it doesn't make it incorrect. That is one of the best things about mindfulness practice. There is no right or wrong, there is just the result. If you can attain a mindful presence within and you are not using a single technique we have listed here, that is fantastic! It is your journey not anyone else's.

Benefits of Guided Meditation

You are most likely here right now because you have heard amazing, life-changing aspects meditation can bring to your life. Whether you are looking to improve your mental health, performance, physical health, or better your relationship with yourself or others; meditation could be the perfect practice for you.

Mental Health Benefits

Unfortunately, there are many individuals who suffer from mental health issues. Whether you are dealing with anxiety, depression, or something along those lines; meditation can help place you in a better mindset when practiced on a regular basis.

Decrease Depression

In a study done in Belgium, four-hundred students were placed in an in-class mindfulness program to see if it could reduce their stress, anxiety, and depression. It was found that six months later, the students who practiced were less likely to develop depression-like symptoms. It was found that mindfulness meditation could potentially be just as effective as an antidepressant drug!

In another study, women who were going through a high-risk pregnancy were asked to participate in a mindfulness yoga exercise for ten weeks. After the time passed, it was found there was a significant reduction in the symptoms often caused by depression. On top of the benefit of less depression, the mothers also showed signs of having a more intense bond with their child while it was still in the womb.

Reduce Anxiety and Depression

In general, meditation may be best known for the mental health benefits of reducing the symptoms associated with anxiety and depression. It was found that through meditation, individuals who practiced meditation such as Vipassana or "Open Monitoring Meditation," were able to reduce the grey-matter density in their brains. This grey-matter is related to stress and anxiety. When individuals practice meditation, it helps create an environment where they can live moment to moment rather than getting stuck in one situation.

While practicing meditation, the positive mindset may be able to help regulate anxiety and mood disorders that are associated with panic disorders. There was one article published in the American Journal of Psychiatry based around twenty-two different patients who had panic or anxiety disorders. After three months of relaxation and meditation, twenty of the twenty-two were able to reduce the effects of their panic and anxiety.

Performance Benefits

When you are able to relax, you would be amazed at how much better your brain will be able to function. By letting go of stress, you leave room for positive thoughts in your head and will be able to make better decisions for yourself. It's a win-win situation when you can improve your mood and your performance simply from meditation.

Better Decision Making

A study done at UCLA found that for individuals who practiced meditation for a long time, had a larger amount of gyrification in the brain. This is the "folding" along the cortex, which is directly related to processing information faster. Compared to individuals who do not practice meditation, it was found that meditators were able to form memories easier, make quicker decisions, and could process information at a higher rate overall.

Improve Focus and Attention

Another study performed at the University of California suggested that through meditation, subjects are able to increase their focus on tasks, especially ones that are boring and repetitive. It was found that even after only twenty minutes of meditation practice, individuals are able to increase their cognitive skills ten times better compared to those who do not practice mindfulness.

Along the same lines, it's believed that meditation may be able to help manage those who have ADHD, or attention deficit hyperactivity disorder. There was a study performed on fifty adults who had ADHD. The group was placed through mindfulness-based cognitive therapy to see how it would affect their ADHD. In the end, it was found that these individuals were able to act with awareness while reducing both their impulsivity and hyperactivity. Overall, they were able to improve their inattention.

Relieve Pain

It has been said that it's possible that meditation could potentially relieve pain better when compared to morphine. This may be possible due to the fact that pain is subjective. There was a study done on thirteen Zen masters compared to thirteen non-practitioners. These individuals were exposed to painful heat whilst having their brain activity watched. The Zen masters reported less pain, and the neurological output reported less pain as well. This goes to show that pain truly is a mental aspect.

Along the same lines, mindfulness training could also help patients who have been diagnosed with Fibromyalgia. In one study, there were eleven patients who went through eight weeks of training for mindfulness. At the end of the study, the overall health of these individuals improved and reported more good days than bad.

Avoid Multitasking Too Often

While multitasking can seem like a good skill to have at some points, it's also an excellent way to become overwhelmed and stressed out. Unfortunately, multitasking can be very dangerous to your productivity. When you ask your brain to switch gears between activities, this often can produce distractions from your work being done. A study was performed on students at the University of Arizona and the University of Washington. These people were placed through eight weeks of mindfulness meditation. During this time, the students had to perform a stressful test demonstrating multitasking before and after the training.

It was shown that those who practiced meditation were able to increase their memory and lower their stress while multitasking.

Physical Benefits

While mental improvements are fantastic benefits of meditation, physical benefits can help motivate individuals to begin meditation as well. Unfortunately, the standard of health is to turn to medication. If you are an individual who hates popping pills for every issue you have; meditation may be just what you need to help improve your health.

Reduce Risk of Stroke and Heart Disease

It has been found that heart disease is one of the top killers in the world compared to other illnesses. Through meditation, it's possible you could lower your risk of both heart disease and stroke. There was a study done in 2012 for a group of two hundred high-risk people. These individuals were asked to take a class on health, exercise, or take a class on meditation. Over the next five years, it was found that the individuals who chose meditation were able to reduce their risk of death, stroke, and heart attacks by almost half!

Reduce High Blood Pressure

In a clinical study based around meditation, it was also found that certain Zen meditations such as Zazen, has the ability to lower both stress and high blood pressures. It's believed that relaxation response techniques could lower blood pressure levels after three short months of practicing. Through meditation, individuals had less need for medication for their blood pressure! This could potentially be due to the fact that when we relax, it helps open your blood vessels through the formation of nitric oxide.

Live a Longer Life

When you get rid of stress in your life, you may be amazed at how much more energetic and healthier you feel. While the research hasn't been drawn to a conclusion yet, there are some studies that suggest meditation could have an effect on the telomere length in our cells.

267

Telomeres are in charge of how our cells age. When there is less cognitive stress, it helps maintain telomere and other hormonal factors.

Relationship Benefits

There are some people who are looking for a little bit more peace in your life. In the world we live in today, times can be very trying. There are constant deadlines, bills to pay, people to deal with; but now is the time to look at stressors in your life under a different life. Through meditation, you can become a more caring and empathetic individual to create a more peaceful life for yourself.

Improve Positive Relationships and Empathy

When we undergo stressful situations with obnoxious people, it can be very trying to remain empathetic. There is a Buddhist tradition of practicing loving-kindness meditation that may be able to help foster a sense of care toward all living things. Through meditation, you'll be able to boost the way you read facial expressions and gain the ability to empathize with others. When you have a loving attitude toward yourself and others, this helps develop a positive relationship with them and a sense of self-acceptance.

Decrease Feelings of Loneliness

There are many people who are not okay with being alone. Often times, we try to fill our time with activities so that we are never alone with ourselves. The truth is, it can be healthy to spend some time with yourself so that you can self-reflect on your life choices. In a study published in Brain, Behavior, and Immunity, it was proven that after thirty minutes of meditation per day, it was able to reduce individuals' sense of loneliness while reducing the risks of premature death, depression, and perhaps even Alzheimer's.

Along with feeling less lonely, meditation also opens up new doors to feeling a positive connection to yourself. When you love yourself, and you are happy with your own company, you may spend a lot less time on negative thoughts and feelings of self-doubt; both of which can lead to self-caused stress.

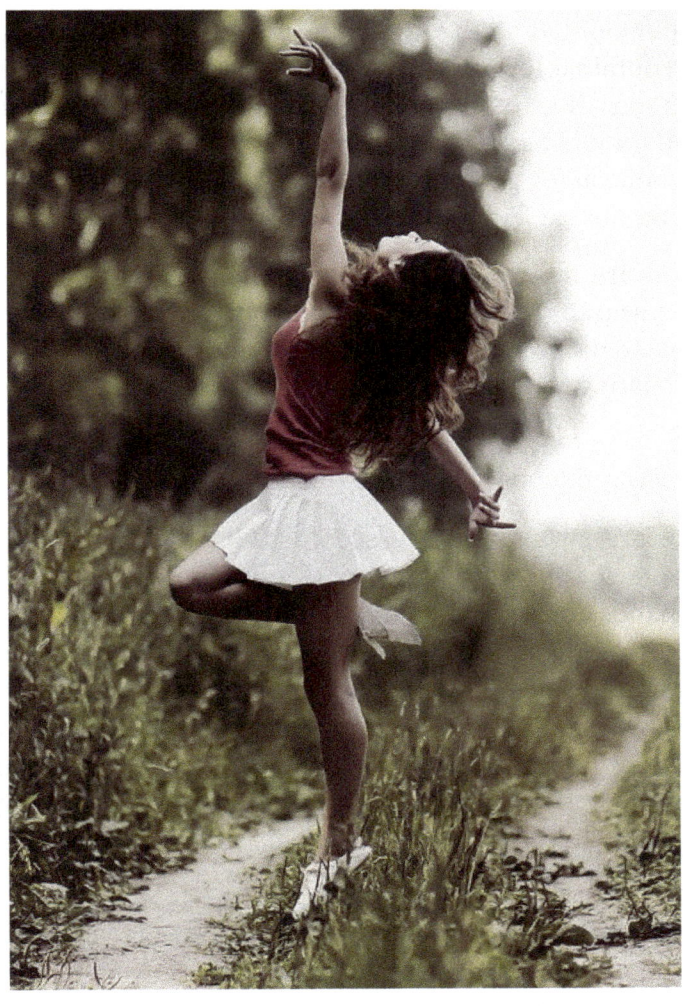

How to Eat with the Help of Meditation

Have you ever asked yourself, when was the last time you went to the market to buy fruits? You go to the market most of the time, intending to buy other foods, but you hardly think of buying fruits. The fruit is very healthy, and they contain lots of nutritional benefits, especially if you are the type of person that loves sweet things. Instead of buying unhealthy things that contain a lot of sugars and calories, you can decide to buy fruits. Fruits add value to your body, and they prevent you from diseases. They contain minerals that your body needs. Now since you know that fruits are beneficial for you, the problem is that most times you tend to forget that you can eat fruits.

So, when you are hungry, you tend to munch on your favorite carbs without even searching for some fruits to eat. So, meditation will help you to be able to differentiate between right and wrong. It will help you to know that eating fruit is beneficial for your body so that you continue to eat fruits.

Avoiding processed foods

Today there are so many processed foods in the market. The food industry is one of the fastest-growing industries today, and as the industry expands, more and more businesspeople are now trying to make money from selling processed foods. New food companies are gaining momentum and are trying to sell fast foods to people. One of the aims of these companies is to stop you from buying fruits that will not be beneficial to you. They are experts at targeting the market. They know that most of the customers in this market have low purchasing power and so they make the food cheap and enticing so that you keep on buying them.

Most of these processed foods contain many chemicals that are harmful to the body, and if you keep eating them, you will only be harming your body. If you want to achieve your ideal weight and live a healthy life, then you need to start avoiding these foods. One of the things that you need to be able to avoid processed foods is discipline. And discipline will help you to be able to make the right decisions on what you should consume and what you should not consume.

Avoiding carbs

Your meal requires just a small portion of carbohydrates, but most times, you tend to consume carbohydrates as your main meal, which then makes you gain weight. One of the major purposes of consuming carbohydrates is to give you energy.

However, when you eat them in excess, not all of them will be used as energy. Some of them will be stored as fat, and they will only make you add weight and they tend to cause sicknesses such as cardiovascular disease. So, if you want to avoid weight gain and such diseases, then it's better that you avoid eating large quantities of carbohydrates. Only eat a small portion of carbs. And make sure that you take the recommended portions of food like bread contains addictive substances, and when you eat them, they make you want to continue to eat more of them. And because of that, you will tend to eat much more than your body needs.

Eat only the recommended portion of food

Eating only the recommended portion of food means only eating the quantity of food that is meant for your body, and chronic eating disorder prevents you from doing so. When you have a chronic eating disorder, you tend to consume more food than the required portion, and many factors cause you to do so. When you are under an eating disorder, you have this belief that, if you eat a lot, you will add weight. And because of that, you keep on eating, and eating does not change your body.

Now the same thing can be applied to when you eat less than the required amount of food. It causes a huge amount of harm to your body. Skipping a meal is not good for you as well as eating too much. They are both dangerous to the body. So, the best thing that you can do is to eat the recommended amount of food that is worth it so that you will stay healthy and fit. So, with the aid of meditation, you will be able to focus and eat the correct portion of food that you are supposed to eat.

Consume plant vegetables and green food

271

Now, these foods contain nutrients that are very vital to the body. Most of these plant-based foods contain minerals to help your body function normally and to be able to conduct all the normal body processes. The nutrients in these foods are effective in ensuring that you maintain good health.

It also helps to provide minerals that prevent certain diseases. Some of these minerals help in boosting the metabolic processes that occur in your body. If you have not been consuming plant-based food before, then it is better to start now. Plant-based foods are very important when you're trying to lose weight; they will ensure that you only eat the right portion. If you really want to lose weight, then you should turn to plant-based food. They are very beneficial in the weight loss journey.

Our ancestors ate plant-based foods for a long time, they lived healthily, and we're happy. The paleo diet was eaten during the Paleolithic era. At that time, people eat what they planted or what they hunted. They ate the right type of food and lived a healthy life. So, meditation will help you to know when to eat plant-based food and when to eliminate animal-based foods.

Eat lightly cooked food

Most times you tend to overcook your meal, and when you overcook your meal, it offers no benefits to the body, because all the nutrients in the food get lost because of the overcooking. Foods provide a lot of nutrients when they are eating raw or slightly cooked. It takes discipline to be able to cook your food slightly and not to overcook them. Sometimes you will find out that it is easier to cook food when it is fully cooked, especially with the taste that comes with it. In addition, it seems easier and sweet to consume food that has been properly cooked.

However, this kind of food will not help your body in any way. You should choose either to eat right or to enjoy your meal, and if you want to lose weight, then you should choose to eat right and eat healthily. Eating healthy is fun if you truly want to eat. Meditation will help you to set eating goals that will help you to know when not to overcook your food.

Reduce your sugar intake

Sugar is sweet and enticing, but they make you crave for more. They make you simply want more of them. Most times, you tend to crave to eat something sweet. Now eating something sweet isn't bad, but the problem is the danger that comes with it, especially when you consume them in excess. They can be very damaging to the body, so instead of being converted into energy, they are converted into fat, that is why they are very dangerous to the body and when that happens, it leads to further complications in the body.

It leads to diseases like diabetes and tooth problems. And also, they are very addictive, so with discipline, you will be able to avoid sugar, and you'll be able to regulate your sugar consumption. You'll be able to know when to consume sugar and when to avoid it. Meditation will allow you to do that.

You will be able to decide to eat a certain amount of sugar in a day. It will help you to focus on regulating the sugar intake in your body. It will also help you to consume only the sugar that is necessary for the body, so that you will have good health and so that you will have a good body shape.

Avoid overeating

Overeating is one of the very bad habits that you must stop if you really want to lose weight. When you overeat, your body tends to add extra weight. Meditation will help you to be able to practice mindful eating. And mindful eating is essential if you want to maintain good health.

When you practice meditation, you can focus on the food that you are eating. You will be able to know that different foods have different tastes, and some foods will make you full faster at different rates than others. You will be able to analyze how your body feels after eating certain types of food, and you be able to know whether you are satisfied or not so that you will stop eating and not continue to eat. You'll be able to analyze each food and every food that you eat, and the analysis will help you to determine the portion that you should consume every day, depending on the food involved.

As a result, you will able to make well-informed decisions on the foods that you are consuming. You will be able to watch the quantity of food that you eat each day. Now, this might appear like a challenging task to do, but it is not impossible. With meditation, you'll be able to do it. Also, you'll be able to tune your mind into consuming the food that is necessary and ignore whatever is not necessary.

Drink water regularly

Water is essential in promoting good health. People that consume water tend to be healthier and happier than people that don't consume water at all. Also, consuming water will help to prevent you from certain diseases. You can also consume water by eating food that has a lot of water in them like watermelon. The greatest percentage of food is composed of water, so as you consume food, you are also consuming water. You can also decide to drink water with a glass cup. If you're not used to drinking water in the glass cup, then you can start with one or two glasses a day and increase it every day.

If you don't love drinking water, then look for things that will put in the situation to drink water. For instance, you might decide to gift yourself something after drinking a certain amount of water for the day. Drinking water isn't a big deal, and you can train yourself to drink water daily. Meditation will help you to maintain the focus that you need to be able to drink the level of water that you need each day. It will help you to create a plan for drinking water and to stick to that plan.

Benefits of Losing Weight

Shedding pounds can be distressing for some, who are too anxious to even think about achieving their most perfect weight. Well before we understood how undesirable it is, we simply saw having the thin body as absolutely tasteful worth when really our weight remarkably affects both our physical and mental viewpoints. To the individuals who have been hefty for their entire lives, these realities have struck them in negative manners. Presently, getting more fit won't simply balance the feeling of inadequacy they have built up; it will likewise create an uplifting viewpoint towards life. Counseling your own doctor will benefit you, enough to understand that cutting down your weight can be a great deal conceivable. To assist you with getting roused to shed pounds, here are a few benefits to consider.

Benefit One

Stoutness realizes a striking exhibit of burden to the influenced people. It makes some apply more power to move about and do exercises of day by day living. You can't do everything you can do before when you are still inside the typical scope of body weight. At the point when you get thinner, it will empower your body to persevere through basic assignments without feeling any distress. Taking part in a health improvement plan and directing basic activities routinely will help fortify your muscles and will cause you to perform exercises that you can't figure out how to do previously. The example of breathing gets smooth, which permits simpler and improved oxygen conveyance around your body. This experience can be a genuine fortune as you get the opportunity to appreciate life to the fullest with more exercises you can impart to loved ones while never disapproving of, you'll not persevere through each action.

Benefit Two

Heftiness is additionally connected with various types of disease. For ladies, the normal kinds of malignant growth that are connected with being overweight incorporate disease of gallbladder, ovary, bosom, uterus, and colon. This is just intended to keep you educated about the dangers that you hazard yourself into by not lessening weight. Men may likewise create malignant growth because of weight. Men are progressively defenseless to tumors of the colon, rectum, and prostate. It is suggested that you diminish your weight other than maintaining a strategic distance from slims down wealthy in fat and cholesterol.

Large people are likewise exceptionally inclined to malady causing way of life. With unreasonable guilty pleasure to undesirable nourishments and an inactive way of life, you can truly be a possibility for some genuine maladies. Being overweight makes ready to numerous medical issues, in the event that you have conceivably acquired genetic illnesses, at that point it very well may be disturbed. Luckily, slicing off additional loads won't just check numerous wellbeing concerns, however it can likewise assist you with improving and keep up wellbeing status. It might control your standard hypertension, assist you with forestalling heart ailments, keep up your cholesterol level inside range, control rest apnea, and other inconvenience realized by stoutness.

Benefit Three

As it has been accepted that looking great causes you to feel great, sufficiently genuine, when you are fruitful in accomplishing the ideal weight, you will be cheerful as it supports your self-assurance. As you have demonstrated that you can meet whatever objective you may build up, you will be progressively positive throughout everyday life. The penance of getting more fit is unquestionably beneficial in light of the positive picture and upgraded emotional well-being it can give you.

Benefit Four

Decreasing your weight could likewise assist you with preventing rest apnea or lessen it extensively. Rest apnea is a turmoil wherein one quits breathing briefly. It goes on for a concise period and is trailed by overwhelming wheezing. It can cause tiredness and weariness during the day. Overweight individuals are additionally in danger of cardiovascular breakdown because of rest apnea. Expelling those additional layers of fat could help wipe out this issue.

Benefit Five

Diabetes is an intense illness that places one life in danger. Both sort one and type-2 diabetes is related with overweight. For diabetes patients, it is suggested that you take up ordinary exercise and weight reduction diet to control the sugar level of your blood. It will likewise influence the drug that you may be taking at present. You should build your physical exercises. Begin strolling, running, or moving. This will help both in the course of your blood and the decrease of weight.

Benefit Six

At the point when an individual is overweight, knee joints, lower back, and hips apply a great deal to haul him around. It is accepted that these body parts need to apply up to 2-3 times more than typical. This causes pressure and strain in joints. Diminishing your weight will give help to these joints by diminishing the heap they need to convey. This lessens osteoarthritis torment.

Lose fat and addition muscle without cardio. Find the cardio, free fat misfortune exercises utilizing weight preparing activity and stretch preparing to consume fat, dispose of difficult midsection fat, and manufacture muscle.

Benefit Seven

At the point when individuals are discontent with their weight, they are frequently awkward around others. This is an aftereffect of progressing humiliation, uncalled for judgment by society, and obviously, segregation. When one has made progress, and a definitive objective, all these unfortunate propensities, and frustrations will simply vanish. Recover your certainty through having the fortitude to confront anybody, without the sentiment of vulnerability about the appearance, and the manner in which individuals communicate to others.

Popular Meditation Techniques

Mantra Meditation

This is a type of meditation designed to encourage peace, love, and unity, and cultivate and strengthen a sense of compassion. This technique is especially useful if you're having trouble with relationships, or if people are the source of your stress.

1. This meditation works with any position you're comfortable with. Start by practicing breathing meditation for a minute or two. Start focusing on yourself and use positive mantras to send your goodwill towards yourself. Here are some examples of positive mantras:

- let me be safe

- let me be calm

- let me be happy

- let me find peace

You can use as many mantras as you want, and it's up to you whether you say them out loud or just in your head.

2. Keep meditating on yourself for a minute or so. Next, imagine someone you care about, like a lover, a friend, or a family member. Use similar mantras to wish them well and send out your affection and goodwill.

3. After meditating on a loved one for a few minutes, turn your focus to someone for whom you don't have strong feelings, positive or negative, and send them your feelings of compassion or goodwill.

4. The last step is always the most difficult. Visualize someone you have negative feelings for, be it a coworker who rubs you the wrong way, the drunk driver who almost crashed into you on your way home, a group of people whose way of doing things you strongly disagree with, or even the stray cat that sneaks into your house at night and

leaves a big mess everywhere. Meditate on them and use mantras to help you declare feelings of compassion and goodwill for them too. These feelings may not be very genuine at the start, but with repeated practice, that may change.

This type of meditation can bring up strong emotions when visualizing someone you like or someone you don't like. While you shouldn't try to reject those emotions and try to push them away, you shouldn't invite them or dwell on them either. Focus purely on your mantra and the feelings of compassion, unity, and goodwill that you are trying to project.

Body Scan Meditation

This is a form of meditation that focuses on getting to know your body and making sure to relax every part of it.

This meditation is also suitable for any meditation position, but many believe that lying down works best.

1. Spend a minute meditating on your breathing, then turn your focus to your feet. Try to identify all the sensations you can feel in your feet. If you notice any discomfort or tension, try to relieve it. A good way to do this is to imagine breathing air into your feet and letting your muscles slacken.

2. Once your feet are done, move on to your legs. Repeat the process of identifying sensations and relaxing your legs. Keep doing this, gradually moving up your body until you've reached your head. For a short session, you can break your body into fairly large parts, like feet, legs, back, chest arms, hands, shoulders, neck, head. Or you can make it a longer session by doing a more refined scan - toes, feet, ankles, calves, knees, thighs, etc. Make sure you spend extra time on parts of your body that have been under a lot of strain or causing pain recently.

3. Once you've reached your head, meditate on your breathing again for a short while.

4. Repeat the whole process of scanning your body in reverse, starting with your head and moving down to your toes.

Chakra Meditation

Chakras are an important element in managing the flow of energy and are believed to be the points where energy enters the body and is distributed to the rest of your limbs. There are seven chakras in the body located along the spine, directly over the main nerve centers of the nervous system. Each chakra has a specific function and is influenced by related elements in your life. The seven chakras are also each associated with a color, and a mudra and mantra used when meditating. Meditation can be used to open and strengthen the chakras.

First is the Root chakra. It is located at the base of the spine and deals with your natural survival instinct and basic needs. It is blocked by fear and insecurity. The root chakra is associated with the color red, and its mantra during meditation is LAM. Its mudra is the Jnana.

Second is the Sacral chakra, which is located just beneath the naval and manages your reproductive capabilities and all creative elements of the mind. It's associated with the color orange and uses the VAM chakra. For its mudra, rest your hands in your lap with your right hand on top of the left and both palms facing upward. Lift your thumbs and bring the tips together to form a rough circle.

The third chakra is the Solar Plexus chakra and is located directly on top of your belly button. This chakra focuses on both physical and mental power and is important in accepting new experiences. It also helps with digestion. The associated color is yellow, and the mantra is RAM. For the mudra, bring your hands together in front of you between your chest and stomach. Cross your thumbs and turn your hands so your fingertips face forward.

Fourth is the Heart chakra, which is located in the center of your chest. It's strongly connected to your heart and deals with emotions, specifically feelings of love and affection, and healing. The mantra is YAM, the color is green, and for the mudra you use the Jnana, but rather than resting on your knee, your right hand is held over the physical location of the chakra.

Fifth is the Throat chakra which is located in the throat and deals with honesty and communication. It's associated with the color blue and uses the HAM mantra. The mudra is similar to the one used with the Sacral chakra, but rather than resting your hands-on top of each other to form a bigger, more exact circle.

The sixth chakra is the Third-Eye chakra. It is located in the center of your forehead, and deals with intuition and understanding, both mundane and spiritual. It is also believed to be connected to psychic abilities. It is represented by the color purple and uses the SHANG mantra. For the mudra, bring your hands together in front of your chest. Bend all your fingers except the middle fingers and thumbs down at the first joint and press them to their counterpart on the opposite hand. Straighten your middle fingers and press their tips together. Relax your thumbs.

Finally comes the Crown chakra. It's located at the very top of your head and connects you to the divine energy of the universe around you. This chakra is naturally blocked, and opening it is nearly impossible, and takes years of meditation. It is associated with white or gold and uses the OM mantra. To use the mudra, bring your hands together in front of your stomach and interlace your fingers. Press your palms together and straighten your pinkies so they're pointing upward.

Normally your chakras are blocked, and the flow of energy within your body is inhibited. Most people go through life not realizing their chakras are blocked, and it doesn't cause too much of a problem for them. Opening the chakras, however, can have an incredible effect on your mind and body, and improve your life. Meditating to open your chakras can initially be done in two ways: either by meditating on one chakra individually, or by meditating to open all of them in one session. This meditation works best with seated meditation or lying down.

For meditating on all chakras:

1. Start with your root chakra, and visualize energy moving from the earth into your feet, up your legs, and into the root chakra. Imagine the energy forming a red light beginning to spin, faster and faster, on the area where your root chakra is located. It doesn't matter in which direction the light spins.

2. Once you have that image settled in your mind, meditate on the elements in your life that block this chakra - things that you fear and make you feel uncertain and unsafe. Accept these fears and try to let them go. Use the mudra and mantra for the root chakra if you want.

3. Let the energy from your root chakra move up along your spine into the sacral chakra, turning from red to orange, and let it spin there. Make sure you visualize the energy spinning in the same direction as the previous chakra. Switch over to the mudra and mantra for this chakra and meditate on what might be blocking this chakra, like changes you are unwilling to accept, or creative blocks in your daily life.

4. Working your way up your spine, repeat this process for each of the chakras, using the associated color for your visualization of each, as well as the correct mudra and mantra. Here is what you should meditate on for each chakra:

• Solar plexus - things that throw you off balance, and new experiences that you are having trouble accepting and coping with.

• Heart chakra - relationships you are having trouble with or have lost, and problems impeding your physical and spiritual healing.

• Throat chakra - lies you've told to yourself, and troubles you have communicating with others.

• third-eye chakra - things in your life that keep you from seeing the world clearly. You can also meditate on spiritual matters and any latent psychic talents you may have if you want to develop them.

- Crown chakra - things that bind you to this world and keep you from connecting to higher energies.

   5. Once you've meditated on the last chakra, visualize the energy flowing out of your body, moving back down your spine through each of the chakras, until it finally leaves through your legs and fades back into the earth.

Chakra meditation with crystals is also very easy. If you're meditating on a single chakra, simply hold a crystal that resonates with that chakra in your hands while you meditate. If meditating on all the chakras, lie down and place an appropriate crystal on your body above the area where your chakra is located, placing the crystal for your root chakra on the ground between your legs and the crown chakra just above the crown of your head. Feel the energy of each crystal as you meditate.

Meditation for a Healthy Diet and Body Image

People always associate bodyweight genes or external factors like, eating habits, available food at one's disposal, or emotional stress. People do try to escape the fact that they are responsible for their eating choices and the quantity of the food they eat. This makes it easy to go back to our original poor eating habits even after we have started meditation. However, through meditation, we get to understand our role and contribution to our own journey to weight loss. Changing one's eating habits and patterns is not an easy step and requires a lot of patience, motivation, and focus. Always surround yourself with people who can motivate you to make healthier choices. We need not blame our genes but try to work on making better health choices.

Helpful Tips to Food and Meditation

- Go slow with your meals, put more emphasis on chewing very slowly, and know the taste of each bite. Treat the moment as if you will describe to someone exactly how the food tastes like. By doing this, it helps you keep the focus on the food you eat and appreciate different taste, even the most unpleasant.

- Create a mealtime and adhere to it. Avoid eating when you are doing something else; also, this prevents overindulging and helps you measure the quantity as well as eat to satisfaction and not leisure. Multitasking, as you eat, can lead to overeating or indulging in unhealthy foods.

- Respond to hunger and satisfaction. When you are hungry eat do not deny your body food, this also applies to when you are full; you should stop eating. Listen and communicate with your body whatever it is telling you to respond appropriately.

- Know how different kinds of food make you feel. This is after you eat them. This statement mostly responds to questions

284

like, which meal makes you tired or energized? Avoid food that makes you tired since they reduce the body's metabolism.

- Learn to forgive yourself for overindulging even when you are not hungry. The food that you ate because you wanted to but made you tired just forget about them and continue with the food that keeps you energized. Understand that you are not perfect and are bound to be tempted to eat the foods you don't want to eat. When you give in to temptation, forgive yourself, and move on.

- Spend time and make responsible food choices, always plan for the kind of foods you'll eat in advance. If you can't do this all the time, make a weekly or daily meal plan.

- Acknowledge your food cravings. By doing this, you will be able to resist your craving by understanding that it is reasonable to crave, but you do not have to give in to all types of cravings.

We can design specific techniques and practices concerning mindful eating, meditating, and intuitive eating. By these techniques, we get to have a healthy and productive relationship with regards to food and thereby to eliminate any bad feelings associated with diet and our eating habits. The result of this is healthy weight loss though this should not be the key focus; it should serve more as a reward. If we focus on weight loss as the primary goal, then we may be distracted and not have a focused mind during meditation. When eating, though, you should eat because you are hungry and need to satisfy yourself. Do not eat because you are stressed at work, stressed with family issues, so you need to eat to forget about your stress. Meditation practices help you love your body and be in control of your mind and the decisions you make.

Through meditation, our mind is inclined to a diet that we believe is beneficial to us. Since we will understand that if we lose weight, we will be healthier and more productive. It is good when your mind controls the food you eat. This is because it will even influence your attitude towards that food and help you make healthier food choices. Do not be surprised if the food you used to eat for comfort or that food that always makes you happy suddenly becomes your least favorite food. Once the mind influences the attitude, we start making judgments, which in turn affects our emotions and thus shapes our way of thing.

If meditation is easy, why then do we still not lose weight? If you start meditation for weight loss when your mind is not prepared. Your focus on other things, you will be wasting your time because the chances that you are spending your time is very high.

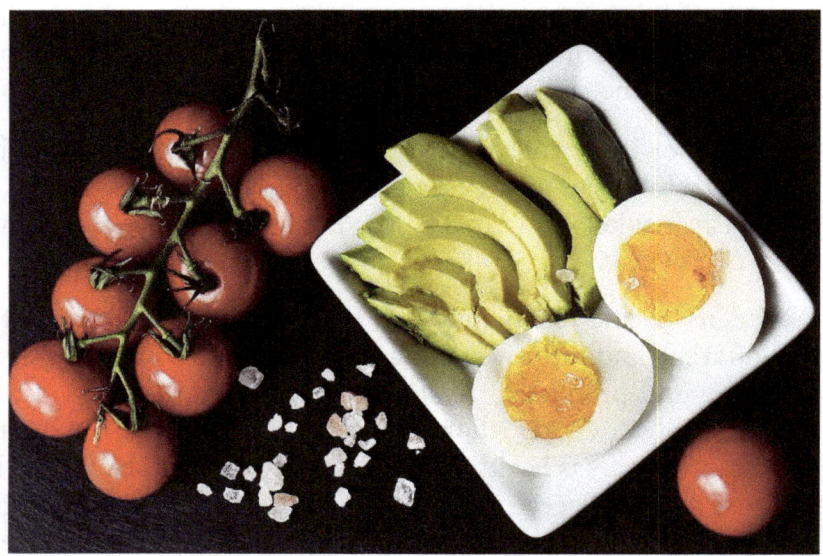

Benefits of Having a Healthy Body

Benefits of maintaining a healthy body

It is important to maintain a healthy body in order to maintain achieve a healthy life. A healthy body enables one to lead an active and more productive life, which directly translates to great achievements and also age gracefully. In order to maintain a healthy body, one has to have a healthy diet, subject himself/herself to regular exercises, maintain a stress-free mind, have a quality sleep and also, lead a healthy lifestyle. The following are ten important reasons for maintaining a healthy body.

1. Boosts the immune system

A healthy body means that all the body processes are working at their best, and therefore all required antibodies for fighting illness are produced in enough amounts. This way, the body is able to fight off illnesses and protect the body from getting sick. Even though the body cannot fight off all illness, a healthy body is likely to fight off most seasonal illnesses compared to the non-healthy body. It is advised, however, that if the body's immune system goes down, it is important to avoid consuming alcohol or taking in food and drinks that are sugary as microbes have a high affinity for sugar.

2. Reduces chances of getting any type of cancer

From a biological explanation, cancer is the uncontrolled division of cells due to a mutation of the DNA within cells. DNA is responsible for giving cells instruction on when to divide, how much cells to divide, and also repair cells that need repairing. When the DNA mutates, the cells divide uncontrollably and not perform the required tasks leading to cancer. Causes of DNA mutations are either inherited genetically, biologically predisposed through chemical causing cancer or unhealthy lifestyles like poor diet, smoking, consumption of loads amounts of alcohol, and obesity. Unhealthy lifestyles are the number one cause of cancer. A healthy body contains a normal DNA, which means a controlled cell division and also, proper repair of cells. It is therefore important to maintain a healthy body

3. Increases the body energy level

A healthy body has high levels of energy, which are as a result of the work put in to achieve it. Being healthy means having a healthy diet. A healthy diet means that the body is supplied with the required vitamins, carbohydrates, and proteins required. Exercising makes the body adapt to harsh treatment, and in return, every exercise session leaves the body even stronger than it was before. Enough sleep clears the mind and also gets rid of fatigue. This compilation ultimately translates to the body having high energy levels and more productive.

4. Reduces chances of being infertile

Being overweight or underweight can increase one chance of being infertile. Also, the abuse of recreational drugs and smoking can also contribute greatly to infertility. Being overweight, smoking and consuming loads of alcohol in men reduce the sperm count leading to infertility. Both being underweight and overweight in women also contributes to infertility. All the above stated problems are a result of an unhealthy body. Therefore, eating healthy to avoid underweight, exercising to curb obesity and overweight cases and leading a healthy lifestyle and minting a healthy body can go a long way in the cure for infertility.

5. Prevents stroke and heart related problems

Stroke is where the brain is deprived of oxygen for a while, causing death to its cells. Deprivation of oxygen may be caused by blockage of arteries or rupturing of arteries leading to leakage of oxygenated blood responsible for keeping cells up and running. Among the causes of blocked arteries is due to deposition of fat blocking the proper flow of blood to the brain. Other causes may include unhealthy lifestyles and stress. Heart problems include heart attack and coronary artery disease. Similarly, coronary artery disease is caused by too much cholesterol blocking the supply of blood to the body. A heart attack is the rapture of the coronary artery; it is as a result of the heart pumping blood at a higher rhythmic pressure than the normal one. This creates pressure on the artery causing them to rapture. The best treatment approved by doctors for both diseases is exercising, leading a healthy lifestyle, having enough rest, avoiding stress and also adopting a healthy diet. Doctors stress keeping our bodies healthy as we are able to fight off illnesses like heart problems and stroke among others.

6. Enhances some career choices

Careers like athletics require athletes to maintain healthy living standards and impressive body physique. Athletes are required to adopt a strict diet, exercise regularly, and subject their bodies to enough sleep and, most of all, avoid consumption of recreational drugs as well as too much alcohol if not a small amount. In the entertainment industry too, models and dancers mostly are required to adhere to similar living standards. These healthy standards ensure their bodies are at optimum health and they are able to remain top of their careers.

7. Improves longevity

Study within time has shown that having a healthy body ensures one to achieve a long life. Exercising as little as twenty minutes a day reduced the chances of one suffering a premature death. Healthy adjustments like proper diet are also essential in achieving a long life. The healthy body even at an older age also means that one is able to carry out tasks which would have been hard if they were unhealthy or dead. It also means that one is able to enjoy more time with family. Grandparents get a chance to see and bond with their grandchildren all because of maintaining their bodies at healthy levels

8. Helps control body weight

A healthy body is a state acquired after proper care of the body and exercises. Even without trying to lose weight, healthy living standards will ultimately lead to a healthy body weight. A weekly schedule of a few hours of exercise and eating right will go a long way in maintaining a healthy body weight. The body will have a strong immune system, prevent heart diseases and also spike the body energy level all as a result of a healthy body

9. Improves moods and feelings

A study has proven that exercising our body leaves our bodies relaxed and happy also. This is a result of the release of brain cell chemicals called endorphins. Exercising also ensures that one achieves an athletic physique, which means that one will have improved physical appearances leading to improved self-confidence. We live in a world of constant disappointments and tragedies. It is important to keep out bodies at most health for improved emotional balance and also maximum cognitive functions

10.   Helps manage diabetes

There are two main types of diabetes, type one where the body insulin producing cells are attacked by the body itself, and one has to live on insulin shots all his/ her life and type two diabetes where the body is unable to absorb the sugar in the blood and convert it into energy for the cells. Type one diabetes is a result of poor health living standards, lack of exercises and having a poor diet. Early stages of diabetes like Prediabetes and also gestational diabetes can be controlled by a proper diet and exercise. Maintaining a healthy body will mean that the body will be able to control body insulin balance and reduce fatalities caused by Diabetes like blood pressure, heart attack, kidney failure and hardening of blood vessels

11.   Improves the brains memory

A healthy body constitutes a healthy diet; a healthy diet comprises of all the food nutrients. Among these nutrients are vitamins. Vitamins preferably C, E, D, Omega 3, fatty acids and flavonoids are essential in developing a brain with a good memory. A healthy diet also helps fight off dementia and decline of cognitive functions. Dementia is the loss of memory, effects on the ability to speak, think or even solve a problem. Eating healthy will help reduce dementia that which is not caused by physical injury on the brain.

12.   Strengthens both the bones and the teeth.

Maintaining a healthy body helps improve the strength of teeth and bones. It is advisable to consume dairy products for calcium three portions a day. One is also required to subject the body to physical exercises, and the most preferred one is lifting weights. A proper diet is essential as well. One is required to consume meals rich in calcium and magnesium for stronger teeth and bones. Many kinds of cereal contain calcium while magnesium is abundantly found in legumes, nuts, whole grains and seeds

13.   Boosts self-esteem

Among reasons for having low self-esteem is having an unhealthy body. We live in a world of diversity and one that is rich in different tastes in fashion. Often everyone wants to look good, but at times our bodies often fail us, and this can be bad for our self-esteem. However, this can be changed, and our esteem boosted within no time. A proper diet would be a good start accompanied by regular body exercises and maintaining a healthy mind through rest and controlling what we think. Results take time, but eventually, one achieves a healthy body. This is more like killing two birds with one stone as one is able to boost their self-confidence by enhancing appearances and also achieve a state of a healthy body through having a healthy body.

14.   A Healthy body improves better sleep

Often people with unhealthy bodies go through a lot of difficulties when sleeping. They often sweat a lot in cases of obesity and even find difficulties breathing when asleep. Healthy people sleep well and find no difficulties breathing when sleeping. Subjecting the body to exercises ensures the body process work right, and it burns off excess fats causing sweating during the night. Eating right and avoiding abuse of drugs and alcohol also helps achieve a healthy body. A healthy body, in turn, leads to sound sleep

Without a shadow of a doubt, we can comfortably conclude that maintaining healthy bodies is of great importance. A healthy body comes with so many advantages and as above explained it is very easy to achieve a healthy body. One is only required to adopt a healthy diet. Watch what he eats and constantly exercise, at least some few hours in a week. Exercises maintain a healthy weight and also subject our minds to relaxation and happiness. Having enough sleep and rest will do the brain so much good. It is also advised that we lead a healthy lifestyle. Abuse of recreational drugs and overly consumption of alcohol is discouraged. These drugs are fatal to our bodies. The bottom line is that our bodies are our responsibilities, and having a healthy body is a necessity in this age and time.

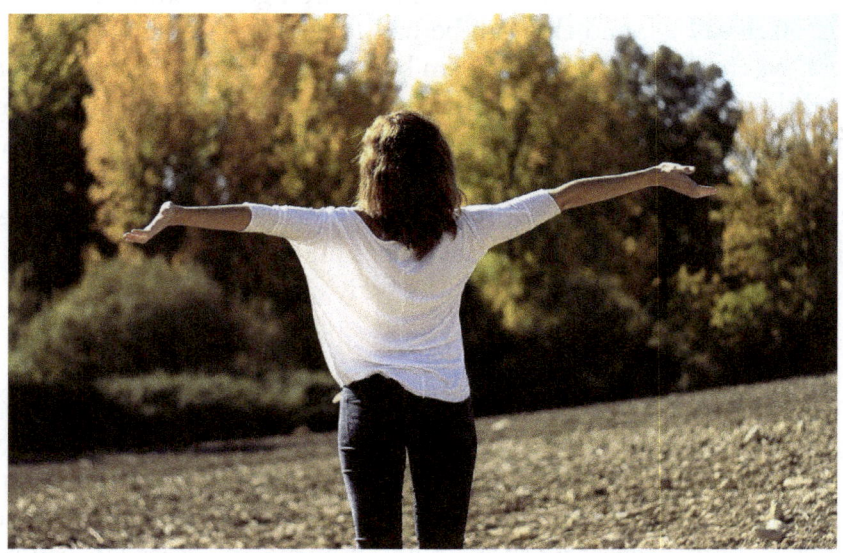

Methods of Meditation

Today's world is just so fast-paced that it feels like we have no time to slow down, relax and be calm. Even when we go on holiday, we take over the office and work in our heads, worrying about the next board meeting, a disgruntled client, or where the next deal comes from.

We think we're happy and calm, but within our minds, there are many hidden stresses, fears, worries and thoughts going deep. When we don't take time to relax and quiet the inner noise consciously and intentionally, tension will build up and inevitably affect the quality of our lives, and how we deal with people around us.

It needn't be like this. Meditation practice will allow us to calm down and get still. It helps our mind to get concentrated and relax, helping us to cope with all the everyday stresses of a hectic life.

Meditative Advantages.

A lot of people have various reasons to meditate. When you are contemplating, what was your reason to meditate? To an outsider, if you meditate what they see you do is sit down, maybe cross-legged on the floor, staring at a point in the distance or sit with your eyes closed.

Meditation is some mental activity that has significant health benefits both for the mind and the body. Meditation can help relax the mind, establish a more concentrated state and enhance the functioning of the brain.

Medical evidence suggests that meditation practice appears to elicit a level of physiological relaxation: decreases in blood pressure, slower heartbeats and faster breathing, and other biochemical improvements can occur as well.

1. This reduces the effects of many chronic illnesses, such as heart disease, cancer and diabetes.

2. Helps and soothes chronic pain, anxiety and migraine.

3. Meditation helps improve the role of the immune system and also prevents binge eating.
4. The asthma attacks offer considerable relief.
5. Reduces lactate in the blood, minimizing depression and anxiety.
6. Meditation has been documented to also help in lowering cholesterol.
7. Reduces muscle tension, and the nervous system is relaxed.
8. It assists in building self-confidence.
9. Helps monitor an aggressive mind.
10. Increases synchronization between brain waves.
11. Removing unhealthy habits helps.
12. Assists in the creation of intuition, imagination and concentration.
13. Improves the ability to remember and improves memory retention.
14. Enhances sleep habits and assists in eradicating insomnia.

Meditation is the process of thought intensely for a while or relaxing one's mind. This can be done in silence or with the assistance of singing and is done for a variety of reasons, ranging among religious or spiritual motives to a way to induce relaxation.

Meditation has in recent years grown in popularity in our modern, eventful world as a way to relieve stress. It has also emerged scientific evidence that meditation can be a valuable tool in the fight against chronic diseases, including depression, heart disease and chronic pain.

This ancient custom has many different aspects to it.

How can I remain motivated to lose weight?

The most critical aspect of creating relentless and virtually infinite inspiration is linked with all the reasons you want to lose weight.

- Keep in mind the broader sense of weight loss for you, like your health needs or how it can positively affect you every day, and the people around you, such as your family and close friends.

- Focus on clear, observable, achievable, timely and practical objectives. Make short but attainable goals first to find enjoyment and fulfilment in constant progress towards achieving long-term goals of weight loss.

- Have a clear, rational mind of not being too easy or too hard on yourself to reach the objectives by keeping the confidence and frustrations going far away.

- Find people around you with the same drive as you do, and you are constantly encouraged and challenged to continue pushing for similar goals.

When you can keep these continually in mind, you can find that you will feel more motivated and determined to work through obstacles and circumstances toward achieving your long-term goals.

Methods of meditation

Conscious Meditation. It's easy to get caught up in a loop of spinning thoughts — starting to think about a laundry list of activities to do, ruminating about past events, or potentially future situations — and practicing mindfulness may help. Yet what exactly is attention? It can be described as a mental state that requires being fully engaged on "the now" so that, without judgment, you can understand and acknowledge your thoughts, feelings and sensations.

Mindfulness meditation is a form of mental preparation that helps you to slow down thoughts of running, let go of anger and relax both your mind and body. Mindfulness methods can vary, but a meditation on mindfulness generally involves breathing exercise, mental imagery, body and mind awareness, and relaxation of the muscle and organ. Practicing meditation with mindfulness does not require props or planning (no need for candles, essential oils or mantras, unless you enjoy it). To get going, all you need is a comfortable sitting spot, three to five minutes of spare time and an attitude that's free of judgment.

Mindfulness meditation is the method of having your thoughts fully present. Knowledge involves being mindful of where we are and what we do, and not being too sensitive to what is happening around us.

One can do reflective meditation anywhere. Some people like to sit in a quiet spot, close their eyes and focus on their respiration. But at every stage of the day, even when driving to work or doing chores, you can choose to be conscious.

You track your thoughts and feelings while practicing mindfulness meditation but let them move without judgment.

Transcendental meditation. Transcendental meditation is an essential technique whereby an individually defined rhythm, such as a word, sound, or short phrase, is repeated in a particular way. It is exercised twice per day for 20 minutes while sitting comfortably close to the eyes.

The hope is that this technique will allow you to settle into a deep state of relaxation to achieve inner peace without attention or effort.

Directed Meditation. Directed meditation, often also referred to as guided imagery or visualization, is a meditation technique in which you create mental images or scenarios that you find calming.

Vipassana Meditation. Vipassana meditation is an ancient form of Indian meditation which means seeing things as they are. More than 2,500 years ago, it was taught in India. Conscious meditation movement has origins in this practice in the United States.

The purpose of meditation with vipassana is self-transformation through the examination of oneself. The sustained interconnectedness leads to a happy account filled with love and compassion.

Vipassana is usually taught during a 10-day course in this tradition, and people are expected to follow a set of rules all the time, as well as for abstaining from all intoxicants, telling lies, cheating, sexual activity, and killing any animals.

Meditation Yoga. The yoga practice has its roots in ancient India. There are a wide variety of yoga classes and styles, but all include performing a series of postures and guided breathing exercises designed to encourage flexibility and relax the mind.

The poses require balance and attention, and practitioners are encouraged to concentrate less on distractions and remain more at the moment.

Which meditation style you choose to try, depends on several factors. When you have a health problem and are new to yoga, tell your doctor what method would be right for you.

Ways to Promote Meditation into Your Life.

Treat yourself to ice cream? Are you stuck in the motorway? A friend in wait? Here's how to make these moments a meditation.

Which one considers harder: in sleep, taming your monkey mind or making extra time only to sit still every day? Either way, fear not: by merely integrating meditation into your daily activities, you can quickly reach a calm state of mind.

1. Do that you want to do. If it's hiking, walking, cooking or painting, while we concentrate wholeheartedly on our favorite things, time stands still. Mysteriously, our stream of emotions, stories and dramas fall away. Submerge yourself in this One Amazing Thing, and don't pay heed to those pings! Then keep an eye on your feelings. Calmer, then? Feeling happier? Congratulations — you've just completed a meditation on the influence of the present moment. That is so simple.

2. Nurture Nature Yourself. Life is not like a popular dietary supplement, with people happily hiking every day. And almost anytime you go outside, you can quickly practice meditation. As you adapt to the primary rhythms of nature, your breath and thoughts slow down to match the gentle march of Mother Nature.

3. Only making yourself like your ten-year-old self and observing the clouds overhead will transmute stress. Extra credit if you consider heart types blowing down the shadows.

4. Wait not, meditate! You meet a friend, and she is delayed — again. Seek a smartphone meditation instead of wasting time tweeting and texting. Indeed, there's an application for that! Plug your ear buds, and you are all of a sudden, engaged in a 10-minute session that is oh-so-soothing. By the time you're done, bet you your friend arrives — and that you welcome her with a warm embrace instead of the "late-again" eye-roll.

5. Time to Fly. If you're caught in traffic, now isn't necessarily the time to "be one with your fellow riders" and surrender blissfully. You need a serene diversion. Try a mantra meditation set to create super chill music (I am a major DJ Drez fan) or invent your own ("I am love, I am light") and get lost as you walk down the lane.

6. Eat your favorite food Drop-Dead. Step into the kitchen with your oh-so-spiritual self and scoop up a small helping of ice cream or anything tickles your buds. This ancient tradition of mindful eating is both an essential rite of contemplation and a fantastic way of expressing appreciation for our abundance.

7. Meditation, meditation, and yoga and more. Truth: It is the physical poses that allow us to get into that dark, still space in our minds.

What Makes Your Body Gain Weight: Daily Habits

Types of Eating

We eat to survive, and without food, we will die. Our body needs nutrients to function effectively. Eating because one is hungry is different from eating because there is food or one that wants to eat.

We need to train our system in such a way that we eat to curb hunger just the same way we drink water to quench thirst. While food lovers explore different kinds of food, most of them are keen enough to incorporate healthy eating in their diet.

Mindful Eating

This is a framework used to bring back one's relationship with food and eating experiences. In this technique, your presence is vital, and all the senses are engaged. For instance, how the food smells, the taste of the food, how appetizing it looks, and lastly, your body's reaction to the food.

By this, it mean how that particular food made you feel. Mindful eating always incorporates intuitive eating. It makes the body relax and slow down a little bit as we listen to inner cues of real hunger.

Thus, helping us rectify and reduce emotional binge or emotional eating. Mindful eating can lead to weight loss as long as one makes the right food choices. It is a type of eating that is psychologically controlled, and the food portion measured depending on need. In mind eating, it doesn't matter how much food is there.

What matters is the quantity needed at that particular time. Eating thus becomes a response to hunger other than a leisure activity. People who follow this eating method rarely suffer from obesity. They are physically fit and healthy. During eating also there is no rush regardless of whether one is late or not. The chewing is simultaneous and swallowing.

Intuitive Eating

It is a non-diet approach, mind, and body approach to wellness and health. This approach does not encourage dieting but emphasizes listening to the inner body and hunger cues. By trusting our bodies, intuitive healing renews our relationship with food.

Though it does not encourage dieting, it uses nutritional information to make healthy eating choices and habits. By this habit, we, eat because we need to not because we have to, and dietary values are accepted without bias. In this method we rely more on our intuition. Food is used to satisfy a need. Without the inner cue of hunger, no need for food. For those who want to escape the stress of dieting can appreciate this approach since it is effective and practical. There is no connection between emotions and food in this type of eating.

Emotional or Stress Eating

It happens when people start overeating or under food when they are overwhelmed with mixed emotions rather than eating in response to their inner cues. Strong emotions we experience can sometimes prevent us from listening to our physical feelings and thus preventing us from feeling hungry or full.

In such a scenario, food is used as a mechanism of coping, thus reducing the effect of the intense emotion temporarily. This habit is very addictive, and if not controlled, can lead to obesity, rapid weight gain, overeating, guilt, and shame. Stress-related eating disorder, it cannot handle, can make one vulnerable and not comfortable with their body.

This is where meditation plays a significant role because one will be able to handle their stress situation and, therefore, not use food as a coping mechanism.

Stress eating affects millions of people each year, and although not many will admit it can cause food addiction and unhealthy eating choices. As one eats, they believe eating relieve them of stress and often blame other people for their problems. They do not take responsibility for their actions.

They do not see the need to eat healthy because their mind is preoccupied with so many things.

Dieting

Dieting only changes the food you eat for a while and limit your mindset.

Thus, Meditation will help you tap into your inner feelings and respond to your craving with the ability to control yourself.

Not being in a diet also makes you keep your focus because you will be keen on what you eat and how beneficial it is to your body. Meditation for weight loss changes the perception of the mind, which in turn triggers the inner self to respond to the choices and decisions made. Dieting is restrictive and specific on the meals you are to eat.

It challenges the mind to believe that restriction in terms of food is the only path to weight loss. Meditation, however, is a healthy way of letting the mind be free to choose what is best, learn from mistakes, and be able to focus on becoming better. It is possible to gain weight loss once one stops the diet process. It can offer both long term and short-term weight loss needs. However, the disadvantage is you must know the calories to take per serving. If you do not know, you may take less, and your body will be deprived of the needed nutrient.

Tackling Barriers to Weight Loss

There are so many barriers to weight loss from personal, to medical, to support system and emotional health. Meditation, if incorporated, will bring fruitful and healthy results. Dedication to overcome the challenges and to be focused on achieving your goals is significant. There are so many distractions, especially before you start tour weight loss routine.

Always Be Accountable

Once you have decided to commit to meditation to weight loss, don't shy away from sharing your plan with your support system and family. It is to ensure that the people you share with also reinforce the commitment and form part of the support system. That way, they will feel part of the program and give support whenever there is a need. You can also use apps for reminders and timings; this way, you have a backup plan whenever you forget.

You can also use motivational bands whenever you achieve a milestone set. Being accountable makes you enjoy your successes, acknowledge your failure, and appreciate your support system.

People thrive when they feel responsible for something, especially on something beneficial to their well-being.

Be Educated About Weight Loss

As you embark on meditation for weight loss. Be educated about how it works; that way, weight loss will not be a struggle.

You will be able to handle failed attempts as well as appreciate the progress made.

You will be able to know what you have been doing wrong and decide on the best meditation exercise for you.

If you have misleading information, then your general progress may be inhibited

Weight loss need not be too expensive; neither does it require a costly gym membership or enrolment in a costly meditation class. There are various self-practice meditation exercises that you can comfortably do at home. There are various meal plans and diets that may work for others though they may not offer long term solutions or lasting behavior changes. Have the right information that you need. Don't be misled by anyone posing that they are professionals in that field. Also, do not hesitate to do research online and compare notes. From there, you will be able to come back with something that works for you.

Surround Yourself with a Support System

There are people out there who may be ready and willing to help whenever you want to start or even after you have started.

The support system may include your family, colleagues, friends, or social networks. These groups of amazing people may encourage and support you to meet your long-term goal. After you include them in your plan, they will feel accepted, offer opinions, and check on your progress. Analyze how things are going, as well as encourage you to continue taking a little break when necessary.

Your support system should also include professionals in the field who will give sound advice and offer needed support and care.

Relaxation to Promote Physical Healing

Stress is a hormone that exists within us, which can hinder our ability to lose weight. If you want to ensure that you are doing your best to have well-rounded health, then keeping up with your stress is crucial.

Music can be very relaxing on its own. When you pair it with meditation through mindful listening, it will be much easier to stay focused on what you need to do to live a healthy life while being mindful of the most important things for your overall goals.

Cleansing Relaxation Meditation

This meditation is all about focusing on becoming relaxed and cleansed. One of the best ways to achieve this kind of feeling is through the use of music.

Make sure that you are somewhere comfortable. You need to be in a peaceful and distraction-free zone in which you can close your eyes and focus on nothing but feeling the air come in and leave your body.

One of the reasons why we struggle to lose weight is that we are so stressed. Stress can lead to stress-eating and cause your body to hold onto weight that it does not need. Worse, it can alter your hormonal levels.

You are focused now on reducing stress because this means that it will be easier for you to lose weight. There is nothing else that you are concerned other than becoming more relaxed.

You are centered; you are focused. You are in this moment; you are prepared for whatever might come your way. You are not concerned with anything other than relaxing and becoming more peaceful.

Feel it as the music beats to a rhythm. There is a slight beat, no matter what it is that is being played. Everyone who listens to this will find a different meaning to the tunes. Everyone who partakes in the process of listening to cleansing music does so for different reasons.

It will always help everyone to relax. Though we all have different things that we use this music for, it still helps us to become more and more at peace. Calmer and calmer. More and more relaxed.

Start to focus on your breathing now. Breathe along with the music. Count for at least five while you are breathing in and then five as you are breathing out.

Breathe in for one, two, three, four, and five. Breathe out for six, seven, eight, nine, and 10. Feel as you breathe in how the music enters your body. Your body is like a musical song as well. Your heart is like the drumbeat that is always pounding.

Your brain is like the conductor that tells everything how it should sound. Your blood, your muscles, and your organs – they make up the rest of the instruments. Your body is a beautiful chorus, and you are a melody traveling through life.

You are a perfect being, relaxed, calm, and at peace. You are one with the earth. You are one with the music. You start to feel it come in and out of your body.

This music can change the way you feel. This music is in control of your emotions. It will affect the way you operate.

It is helping you to feel better and more relaxed. It is bringing you closer and closer to being at peace. It is bringing you closer and closer to being centered and focused.

You are feeling lighter and lighter, and the stress is drifting away. As soon as you start to let go of stress, you will start to release yourself from the heavy weights that are keeping you back. The quicker you focus on peace, the more weight you will lose.

Each time you let go of stress, you are letting go of some of your weight. Every time you focus on being more at peace, you are feeling healthier and healthier.

You feel it as the music spreads to every part of your body. It starts in your mind. It stimulates your brain so that you are focused on relaxing and nothing else at that moment.

It soothes your heart. It reminds you that you are not alone. It makes you feel better, and that spreads everywhere else.

The music keeps you motivated. It keeps you cleansed.

Cleansing is an important part of your weight-loss journey. Your body is always working to clean itself. Your body is focused on how it can rid itself of toxins and bring in the things that are good for it. Your breathing is one way that your body is consistently working to cleanse itself.

Your body is always cycling in new air and getting rid of the old. It does the same thing with food as well. It brings in new minerals and nutrients and gets rid of the toxins that it does not need. You drink water to help cleanse your body. It is always working on its own to keep you as cleansed as possible.

The cleansing processes help you to feel more at peace. You feel like a new person. You are constantly given second chances. It is never too late to start over.

You are feeling your body become more and more cleansed now. You are feeling lighter and lighter, more relaxed. You are becoming a new person. You are starting over. You are starting fresh. You are relaxed. You are focused. You are at peace.

Affirmations for Positivity

I am a strong independent person. I do not need to depend on anyone. I am able to take care of myself. I am worthy of everything that comes my way. I understand how to get the things that I want from life. I am completely aware of the things that I am in control of. I'm not afraid of the things that are outside of my control.

I am a capable human being who can achieve anything I set my mind to. I will not let the fear of failure hold me back. I understand that sometimes, failure is a part of the process. I am aware of how to use my mistakes to improve as an individual. I do not need to depend on anybody else for my own happiness. I do not place blame on other individuals for my own mistakes. I do not blame anyone else for the bad things that have come into my life. I am aware of the way that other people might influence certain things in my life, but I am not going to blame them for these things.

I understand what I have to do to achieve the things that I want. I am a motivated person. I am able to motivate myself to get things done. I do not look for any outside sources of motivation. I have the ability to self-reflect and motivate myself from within. I will always honor myself and do what I can to look out for me.

I will always respect myself and the goals I set so I can achieve the things that I want. I know how to set goals and my mindset to be a happier and healthier person.

I am somebody who is actively committed to living a better and healthier life. I am always going to look for methods to improve my life. I will always seek out the moments that make me happier.

I am dedicated to doing the right thing. I am focused on getting the things that I want from this life because I know what I deserve. I am not afraid of being an individual who is not going to get the things that I want. I know exactly how to get the things that I desire the most. My ideas are clear, I have clear and realistic goals, I also have realistic expectations for the things that I will get from this life.

I do not hurt myself. Once I do not achieve a goal. I do not punish myself just because I don't get something that I wanted. I do not hurt myself because I am not happy with who I am. I only love myself. I love the person that I am. I use constant compassion to build myself up. I'm able to self-reflect in a healthy way.

I am aware of my flaws, but I do not beat myself up over them. I know the things that I need to work on. I understand my weaknesses, but I do not let these define me as somebody weak. I know how to change my life in order to get things that I want. I will not let these weaknesses hold me back.

I am aware of these weaknesses and I am ever vigilant of working on them. I understand my flaws and recognize that they make me a unique and interesting individual. I have my own thought processes that are very important to the creativity and uniqueness that I exude.

I let go of all my negative feelings, and instead replace them with positive thoughts. I am able to self-reflect on my negative thoughts in a healthy way, and make sure that I turn them around. I know how to seek out the positive and everything that comes my way. I am aware of the way that I can switch a negative perspective and turn it into a positive one. I choose to be positive every day. I understand what a privilege it is to be able to think within the full scope of your mind. I understand there will still be some days where I can't think positively, but I'm going to commit myself to always trying my best.

I let go of the negative thoughts and emotions of the past. I do not keep myself attached to the toxic mentality that has kept me chained back before. I embrace positivity, and I'm not afraid to be a happy person. I recognize that I am allowed to be happy. I am aware that it is okay for me to be positive. Just because other people aren't positive does not mean that I am not allowed to be.

I can be happy. I will be happy. I am happy. I am comfortable with the person that I am. I am happy and grateful for my body. I understand that I could change things if I wanted to, but I am learning to accept me for me. I do not wish to be anybody else. I hope to change things for the better, but I still appreciate my unique characteristics. I admire other people, but I do not emulate them. I am myself. I am an individual. I have my own important character.

I am aware of all the things that I want to change about myself. I only have realistic expectations and look to change myself for the better. I am grateful for who I am. I am appreciative of the experiences that I have had because they have shaped me into the person I am today. I accept everything that has happened to me, because if not, then that would mean that I might not be the same person. I still have things to work on, but I am appreciative of the character that I have right now.

Conclusion

You have learned a lot of things in this guide. You know how to release your anxiety, how to meditate properly, what the most efficient affirmations are. You can do miracles if you use these techniques properly.

The objective of this guide is to initiate you into a world of losing weight by using affirmative sentences or rather words. In this world, everyone wishes to be happy. Losing weight is just one way to reclaim your happiness back, especially if you have a more significant body. The presence of a right body image is the key to a happy life.

To achieve much in this process of weight loss, you need to embark on areas that give you a clear view of affirmations. Remember, affirmations are just phrases that are highly powerful and lead to positivity in life. By applying these affirmations, be sure that you will be able to stay focus, positive, and relaxed. There are several affirmations that you need to choose from. Try picking the ones you can manage and start your daily routine of making them permanent. Your weight will reduce tremendously.

This guide also aims at making you stay positive about yourself. That's, it indulges you in the world of motivation. Motivational affirmations, therefore, help you in achieving this ultimate goal, thus resulting in a more positive life with lots of happiness and relaxation.

It is now very essential for you to lead a perfect life, free from negativity and obesity. This vital life involves life filled with happiness and morale to live happily and positive. All these results in peace of mind, thus making sure that your inner soul is having elements of blessings. For you to experience all these, you need to get affirmative self-control actions. It will enable you to control everything surrounding you.

When you first meditate, expect hesitation. Expect thoughts to be more important than letting go of them because it's something that you are not accustomed to. The best thing is that if you do it on a daily basis and it becomes a habit rather than taking a lot of effort, then you will learn from this that your body and mind have accepted this road in life and your subconscious mind has registered it as a habit that you don't need to plan all the time. You will really find it as natural as breathing and may even find yourself using mindfulness in all kinds of activities during the course of your life. It's okay to do that because all of the time that you are practicing mindfulness, you are telling those negative thoughts that you have no place for them in your life, and your mind switches over to seeing the cup half full instead of feeling that it is half empty.

Last but not least, this guide consists of various aspects of life that you should follow no matter what. It is through this that you can stay put and straightforward about your personal life and keep at bay every detail of obesity.

Meditation for Weight Loss is, therefore, a manuscript that acts as a guideline in reducing your weight. Your work is to follow it very keenly so that you achieve every detail written here. You should know how best you can make smart goals that can be easily achievable. Without this, then your world is doomed, and you will end up living a life full of frustrations and pain. So, the best way you should follow here is to handle this guide with great care and use every part in fulfilling your dreams of losing weight.

CPSIA information can be obtained
at www.ICGtesting.com
Printed in the USA
BVHW090339190221
600496BV00008B/587